Arthritis Wise

Discover The Causes
Restore Your Health

Ivan Cocks

Published by: Help Thank You LLC, Atlanta, GA 30092
Made in the USA and printed by CreateSpace
Copies of this book are available on Amazon.com and other retailers

All author and publisher references have been placed in the References and Bibliography section towards the end of the book. Every effort has been made to give credit where due: with full mention of published materials so as not to infringe copyright in any way.

Regarding the verses used in Chapter 30 *Red Flags From The Bible,* the following permission is gratefully acknowledged: "All scripture quotations in this publication are from the Good News Translation in Today's English Version- Second Edition Copyright ©1992 by American Bible Society: Used by Permission."

CONTENTS

Disclaimer   i

About The Author   iii

Prologue   v

Dedication   ix

Foreword   xi

Acknowledgments   xv

Introduction   xvii

Getting Sorted   xxiii

1. Misuse Of Statistics   1

2. Medicine Does Not Know   6

3. What Caused It   9

4. Where Did My Health Go   13

5. Louis Pasteur   18

6. Profit Motive In Selling   22

7. The Road To Discovery   27

8. The #1 Cause Of Arthritis   34

9. The Evidence Is All Around You   50

10. Beyond Absolute Common Sense   56

11. Other Supporting Proof   62

12. Another Cause Of Arthritis   70

13. Chickens And Arthritis   75

14. The Essential Oils   79

15. A Cholesterol Story   86

16. What Aggravates Arthritis   94

17. Heredity Ailments   104

18. Alexander Vindicated   107

19. Harmful Preservatives   112

20. Detrimental To Your Health   118

21. What Is Good For You   131

22. Vitamins And Supplements   144

23. Unpleasant Experiences   160

24. Saving You Money   169

25. Overcoming Stress   172

26. Liberation From Depression   176

27. Eliminating Constipation   181

28. Becoming Slimmerer   184

29. Exercise And Rest   192

30. Red Flags From The Bible   196

31. Worthwhile Research   201

32. Preferred Reading   203

33. Moving Your Goalposts   209

34. The Health Prescription   213

Epilogue   217

References And Bibliography   219

Also Available By The Author   225

DISCLAIMER

**It does not require many words
to speak the truth.**
Chief Joseph

The entire contents of this book—the ideas, suggestions and opinions—are presented for educational and information purposes only. Nothing in the title, on the cover or in the contents of this book is intended to imply a guarantee that arthritis, or any other condition, illness or injury; will be healed or eradicated.

It is important to understand, and to note that the author and publisher is not giving medical counsel; health or any kind of personal advice or diagnosis. Neither is it proposed as an alternative to what has been prescribed for you. Please consult with your medical doctor before you make any changes to your medications, your diet or your style of living. Nothing of what is written is intended to replace the advice of your medical doctor, or the medical expertise and prescriptions you have received, and are receiving.

ABOUT THE AUTHOR

Whatever you do act wisely
and consider the end.
German Proverb

The author practiced Investigative Analysis while a professional employee. In his final position he was Group Industrial Engineer in a listed Corporation where he and his staff were responsible for providing Senior Management with a problem solving capability. The Key Objective being:

To evaluate and develop capital expenditure models for new or existing projects—where necessary to attain savings and increase profits.

To solve major problems and bottlenecks affecting the smooth running of operations at all levels: the emphasis being on improving productivity and profitability.

To provide recommendations for the optimum number of people and equipment requirements in relation to maintenance and production needs: by using the appropriate problem solving and other management techniques.

Executing this function meant detailed studies of factors *'causing'* problems; including a proper liaison with knowledgeable specialists in seeking the most favorable answers—then scientifically examining and evaluating all possible solutions to arrive at the best.

In every situation the initial emphasis was always on pinpointing the *'cause'*—at all times the most challenging part of any assignment!

The author started the first of a series of three small businesses in 1983. He has been continually self-employed, since that initial venture.

He has written this book, in part as if it was to be a report to the Executive Board of a Corporation, say, after having been given an assignment to **establish the causes of arthritis.**

With the overall main objective being to **unearth and report on a cure for arthritis**—*in addition to providing working recommendations for the elimination of the ailment.*

PROLOGUE

The person bringing good news
knocks boldly on the door.
Irish Proverb

You may have seen her?

She is a lady who has such a disability she makes use of a motorized cart provided for handicapped customers in your local grocery store. She buzzes around the store loading her cart, before joining the line at the checkout.

Then, as she gives her payment to the register operator, you can see her hands—all deformed with the telltale signs and effects of severe arthritis. And you may have wondered, "How many are like her—in pain or severely incapacitated such as she?"

Unhappily, there are many. In almost every publication you pick up, you are informed that there are over 20 million people suffering with arthritis in varying stages of pain and disability. And that, for some inexplicable reason, this number is predicted to increase greatly over the next decade or so. In fact some predict the number may almost double!

Sadly, except for the sufferers, no one seems to be alarmed. Doctors and drug companies seem happy to prescribe and manufacture painkillers that may relieve the pain and inflammation. And the sadness of it all is that it is so totally unnecessary—because there are those who have been cured—and who are willing to share their secret.

Better still—these people can point to those doctors and researchers who have helped them to find a new and healthier life. The knowledge of these eminent researchers, which has been acquired over the years, is available in books. Books that somehow seem to have been lost to people and doctors in general. They are there—just waiting to be *found* (much like the Dead Sea Scrolls) and presented in such a way that will bring awareness to the fact that there are tried and tested practices that can change and improve the arthritic's quality of life. In reality there is a veritable treasure waiting to be shared and passed on to mankind.

Maybe you are in the same predicament as the lady driving the cart in the grocery store—or are battling with the early symptoms that have recently afflicted you?

Know you can revive your hope, and to take heart from the research which has shown there are several main causes of arthritis. Because once you become aware of them, you can then make the necessary changes in your lifestyle to avoid these causes. Meaning you can embark upon a plan or regimen to restore your health—and then more importantly: maintaining it to the best of your ability thereafter.

Unfortunately the researchers have stated one cannot take away the disfigurement in the fingers and knuckles if the arthritis is that far advanced—although one can remove the pain and inflammation. And the good news is those ancillary ailments that plague arthritics can be healed.

Things like constipation, leg cramps, insomnia, depression, obesity and other irritating problems.

It is like rediscovering your greatest treasure—your health—and having it restored to you.

DEDICATION

**'Tis afterwards that
everything is understood.**
Irish Proverb

To Don Slater—our mentor in the realization one can search for the knowledge that points to finding the treasure of a healthy body.

And to Peggy—the healed arthritic—who rekindled the spark of hope and enthusiasm in discovering what causes arthritis; and other ailments such as diabetes, cancer and heart attacks.

FOREWORD

Seeing is believing.
American Proverb

It was a memorable meeting with Peggy, the lady in the Dedication above, all those years ago. In fact it is best described as a Copernican moment—because both my wife and I were given the opportunity to discover a new lease on life.

As Peggy spoke, her misshapen hands were clearly visible—the arthritis had left its telltale marks: even though she now claimed to be completely cured. A claim she substantiated by stating her granddaughter, who was a pharmacist, had said she was the only person known to her to have been cured from arthritis.

She was no longer on medication and was now *pain free*— and seeing those misshapen and malformed fingers and knuckles made it easy to believe she had suffered acutely from arthritis in the past.

Prior to our meeting with Peggy my wife had begun to develop excruciating pain in her hips. The pain would normally manifest itself at about 3am in the morning—after which time sleep simply eluded her. The pain had progressed to where it developed even when out walking: often so severely she would need to return home.

For myself, I was developing a *loud cricking* in my knees—that was pronounced as I walked down the stairs. A dull sort of pain would appear from time to time in the right knee.

It was a friend of my wife, who suggested we arrange to visit Peggy, after hearing of the onset of our ailments. She had thought it could be arthritis; telling us Peggy might be able to help because she had been healed from arthritis, and would tell us her story.

So it was we found ourselves there that afternoon. And briefly, here are the salient points from her story:

Peggy had developed arthritis at an early age and had gone from doctor to doctor—but had been unable to find a cure. Rather the malady had become worse and worse over the years; affecting her mainly in her hands, with these slowly becoming disfigured.

Eventually the pain had become unbearable, and being a religious sort of person, she decided to go on a prayer pilgrimage hoping she would be healed. While a healing did not occur, she did however met a woman on the excursion who, after hearing Peggy's reason for the trip, told her how she herself had been cured from arthritis: by following the advice outlined in a certain book.

Consequently, on her return home, Peggy had purchased a copy and affirmed she now owed her healing to those same recommendations and methods as outlined by the author.

Naturally, we also bought Dale Alexander's book—and we too are indebted to him. But as of now there are certain things in the book I would caution against: while highlighting those elements that are exceptional. His findings and theories are supported—and greatly improved upon—by the recent research of eminent doctors and authors whose input seems now to complete the overall total picture.

It is the result of the research by these eminent people that makes it possible to state—if their findings and recommendations are implemented: then perfect health is attainable.

That memorable meeting with Peggy occurred about 16 years ago. It has been a sufficiently long trial period to test and verify the work of these brilliant men and women; along with reading the latest research—and so to be able to say—it is factual, and it works!

Their work and theories are discussed through Chapters one to 34 in the *Getting Sorted*, section of the book.

ACKNOWLEDGMENTS

The best portion of a man's life—his little,
nameless, unremembered acts of kindness and love.
William Wordsworth

As one looks back, you remember those people who were *placed in your path* over a lifetime—people who made it their mission both to educate, and to encourage you to develop an enquiring mind.

Initially, there was Brother Killian who, in middle school taught that—*He who asks a question is a fool for five minutes. He who does not is a fool for a lifetime!* All the way through, to people like Don Slater who reveled in using his brain to find solutions to problems: and who did not stint in passing on this knowledge and experience. Don taught how to be *scientific* in one's approach to solving problems and with regards remaining healthy—making the journey a fun experience.

Space does not permit mentioning everyone: all I can do is say, "Thank you!" in general to all those myriads of kind folk that have passed on their knowledge so willingly down through the years.

I thank my parents who provided for me in more ways than one—and as a consequence from whom I learnt so much.

I thank my wife Judy, for her continual support: and for her assistance with the editing of this book. With great love, she has always gone *more than* an extra mile in her efforts to keep me, and our family, healthy and happy.

INTRODUCTION

Two roads diverged in a wood, and I—
I took the 'one less traveled' by.
And that has made all the difference.
Robert Frost

Individually, we are a tiny part of this huge monolithic human race. Because everyone seems so busy and preoccupied—the person who is ill can tend to feel very lonely at times. It must be especially so for arthritics: and thought of the future may seem daunting when they contemplate the nameless hazards that may lie in wait for them.

What is going to happen to me?

Who will help?

Will there be the finances to pay for unknown and huge medical bills?

Discovering the means to regain health will therefore be an assurance of retaining mobility and happiness. And to discover how to be medication free—means money in the bank, through eliminating those costly expenses.

Not only does this promise a better future for you and your family—but when healthy, fit and joyful you can then be of assistance to others, who are less fortunate.

To bring about this happy state of affairs in your life dictates that a good place to begin is probably by reviewing the adage— *God helps those that help themselves.* And the reasoning behind it was once so aptly explained by a visiting college lecturer, whom we will call B.C. She had been invited to be the main speaker at a high school graduation ceremony. Her sensible advice to the graduating students is worth repeating:

The point she made was that up until that time the students had been under the very close and helpful guidance of their lecturers and parents—who all had done the best they could to prepare them for the future. These people had all shown them what to study and when to study, and where to obtain the relevant information.

But that, as they entered the 'world', many situations were to be placed in their paths where they would find they were ill prepared in knowing how to react and deal with events. With the likelihood they would be on their own without someone showing them what to do.

She gave as an example, that with the current high divorce rate: many of the girls present could one day find themselves as single parents—with all sorts of problems to encounter and overcome.

In a nutshell the guidance she offered was that the more they could learn to *self-educate* themselves, the greater the odds they would survive and prosper. That those students, who could adapt early, by learning to seek out knowledge on their own: would find they were in a position to *help themselves.*

In putting her recommendation into practice, and because it is so relevant to arthritis, an excellent place to begin with the research, or *self-education*, is to consider those ailments chiefly suffered by the Romans at the height of the Roman Empire. They had considered they were very civilized and knowledgeable, with their engineers bringing water to the cities in superb architecturally crafted aqua ducts.

Our own scientists and historians now tell us these same aqua ducts, built to carry their water, were in fact lead lined causing lead poisoning in the population—effectively reducing the overall life span to an average of about 55 years. What compounded the situation was their extensive use of lead in the lining of the vessels employed in the wine making process. A fuller article regarding the Romans and the use made of lead can be found in Wikipedia.org, which is a free online encyclopedia. (ref. 10)

The other effect of the all-embracing use of lead, from the Wikipedia write-up, is that a very high percentage of their people ended up getting gout and serious joint pain in their senior years. It was a widespread malady and one the people as a whole could anticipate they would get in their *old age.*

The reason this is especially relevant to people with arthritis is: it shows very clearly that in the case of the Romans' disabilities there was a *'cause'* which begs the question—what is causing the similar widespread arthritic ailment in our own day and age.

Another period in history which leads one to ask the same question is from the people of Paris about 1860. Because of its importance to our own investigation, and in the case to be presented, a separate Chapter 5 has been devoted specifically to considering the work of Louis Pasteur who worked so devotedly to alleviate the suffering of humanity in his time. As you may undoubtedly already know it revolved around the medical professions insistence it was not necessary to wash your hands before treating a patient.

Because of Pasteur's enquiring mind in searching for the cause in the medical problems at the time, he was later able to go on and produce vaccines for other serious ailments such as anthrax and rabies. The results from which we still benefit today.

The following story is a brief recount of the events surrounding my early introduction to finding the 'cause' in things medical through going to work for Don, a manager in a large corporation, while in my late thirties:

Don had suffered a serious heart attack while in his early fifties. Where he was so fortunate was to be treated by a doctor under the guidance of Professor Possel; who was working on an assignment to improve the electrocardiograph (ECG) machine used by the medical profession in measuring and analyzing patients' hearts. The professor, head of the electrical engineering faculty at his university, had as a result of his work in improving the ECG machine; become deeply involved in researching the cause of heart attacks.

His success at helping Don recover was a definite testimony to the thesis that where there is an ailment—there is invariably a cause. And because of his training in problem solving, it was natural for Don to also become interested in learning the mistakes he had previously made in his life style which had brought about his heart attack: and in how to now fully restore his health.

By going to work for Don I learnt of his previous medical issues and in particular his present studies to improve one's physical condition. His success and common sense approach *rubbed off* and for that I am grateful; as mentioned in the Acknowledgements. It is appropriate to mention that Don lived to well over 80 in spite of his serious heart attack as a younger man.

The purpose of this book then is to highlight the results that encompass the work of pioneers who have blazed a trail, so to speak, in discovering the cause of arthritis: and those others whose labors have lead one to form the opinion you can have perfect health. The foundation is also laid for you to continue with your own self-education and research.

A suggestion, as you begin implementing your new lifestyle, is for you to form the habit of measuring your weight each morning, say, before taking a shower. Find out from your health professional your goal weight for your height and age. Some of the ideas and discoveries put forward will make it easy for you to attain your goal weight—but do not go below it.

Secondly, a good idea is to have a blood analysis done before embarking on any new health regnum, and thereafter have it done as a regular preventive measure? A doctor once advised such an analysis should be undertaken every 12 to 18 months. A blood analysis is *scientific* as it is an actual measurement. It measures cholesterol, the minerals in the blood in addition to things like uric acid. File this analysis along with a record of your blood pressure, for future reference and to monitor your progress.

Thirdly, a simple journal will prove invaluable and is actually essential. It can be a simple inexpensive notebook or a file saved on the *desktop* of your computer. Enter dates and changes you make to diet, medications, supplements and vitamins. Do not rely entirely on memory.

GETTING SORTED

If a man will devote his time to securing facts in
an impartial, objective way, his worries will
usually evaporate in the light of knowledge.

Anon

I keep six honest serving men,
they taught me all I know.
Their names are What and Why and When,
and How and Where and Who.

Rudyard Kipling

Misuse Of Statistics
—Chapter 1

Knowledge is power
but only wisdom is liberty.
Will Durant

In an address to a select group of people, and as an introduction to his talk, Professor Possel made the statement that statistics can very easily be misrepresented in the field of medicine. He used this simple humorous example to illustrate his point: *"If you placed a man in a horizontal position—with his head in a fire and his feet in a block of ice—then on average you could say he was comfortable."*

Continuing, he mentioned that in the 1970's a large number of people had died from heart attacks in New York. When, later it was subsequently discovered that many of the refrigerators in New York had broken down just prior to their deaths: it could easily have been assumed, or claimed, that the cause of death in these instances had been the refrigerators breaking down.

Whereas, in point of fact there had been a severe heat wave in the City causing both the high death rate from heart attack plus the malfunctioning refrigerators.

Erroneous conclusions are so easily arrived at in medicine by considering some facts in isolation: rather than embracing all the overall factors that influence a given situation.

Another example one could use is to say that generally arthritics tend to suffer severely from constipation. Therefore, it could be stated that when one is afflicted with arthritis; that this malady in turn causes constipation. Whereas in fact the thing that is causing the constipation is what is also causing the arthritis.

A.K. told this story many years ago to a group of friends while still at college. He said a team of researchers had gone to Tanzania in East Africa, specifically to establish the reason for the low incidence of tooth decay among the people, and especially amongst children; living in rural areas of the country. Subsequently, during their investigations they discovered the concentration of fluoride occurring in the drinking water of the indigenous people was at rather higher levels than the fluoride in our own drinking water.

Based on that finding they came to the conclusion that the reason for the low incidence of tooth decay was the relatively high concentrations of fluoride in the drinking water. A.K. seemed of the opinion that it was because of this study we now have fluoride added to our own drinking water.

Remaining with those scientists for a moment—*they were guilty of a grave error.* The reason being that because of the isolation of the people in their study: and the lack of infrastructure to supply western type delicacies such as sugar, candy and refined white flour to them—the people in the study did not have access to the very things which we know causes cavities.

A Google search was done to attempt to validate A.K.'s story but was unsuccessful. It seems though, that the introduction of fluoride to our drinking water was based on a similar type study in the USA.

Incidentally, if you Google, *the effects of fluoride in Tanzania's water supply* you will be surprised to discover the serious adverse effects, on the local population's health, of excessive amounts of fluoride in their drinking water. So much so, that much research is presently being undertaken, on an ongoing basis, in an attempt to remove this chemical from the water supply.

Because of the importance of understanding how statistics can be misrepresented in medicine—and so give the incorrect picture: please go to Wikipedia.org (ref.10) and read their article under *Misuse of Statistics.* As a primer here is the introduction from the article:

"A misuse of statistics occurs when a statistical argument asserts a falsehood. In some cases, the misuse may be accidental. In others, it is purposeful and for the gain of the perpetrator. When the statistical reason involved is false or misapplied, this constitutes a statistical fallacy.

The false statistics trap can be quite damaging to the quest for knowledge. For example, in medical science, *correcting a falsehood may take decades and cost lives.*

Misuse can be easy to fall into. Professional scientists, even mathematicians and professional statisticians, can be fooled by some simple methods, even if they are careful to check everything."

The article goes on to explain that statistics can be misrepresented or "fudged" by selective reporting or simply by, in some cases, *the making up of false data.* And it gives a good example of why it is important for the researcher to investigate whether or not the data under review could change from year to year.

Sally Fallon with Mary Enig, PhD, in their book *Nourishing Nutrition* (ref.11 p.15) give an actual real case study of how data was misrepresented; much to the detriment of the population as a whole. They report:

"During the 1940s, researchers found a strong correlation between cancer and the consumption of fat—the fats used were *hydrogenated fats* although the results were presented as though the culprit was saturated fats. Thus, natural saturated fats were tarred with the black brush of unnatural hydrogenated vegetable oils."

Reading stuff like that tends to make one wary—and careful not to believe everything that is presented in the media and in selective advertizing. That is why we are so fortunate in having discovered people who have *gone against the stream* and because of their persistence; have developed solutions to the problem under review.

Briefly, returning to the subject of fluoride in water we note that Sally Fallon, in *Nourishing Nutrition* (ref.11 p.53), does not mince words when she says:

"Fluoridated water should be avoided at all costs. Fluoride is an enzyme inhibitor that contributes to bone loss, bone deformities, cancer and a host of other illnesses."

Medicine Does Not Know
—Chapter 2

Only dead fish swim with the stream.
German Proverb

If you have ever had the opportunity to speak with a person with arthritis, it is almost certain you learnt that the cause of their ailment is unknown to medicine: or rather that is what was told to them. That the cartilage in the joints wears out and that arthritis is something you can expect as one gets older.

Specifically, you may discover they have resigned themselves to the belief *there is no cure.* That the best they can hope for is to try different medications in the hope of discovering one which will alleviate the pain the most effectively—and delay the further degeneration of their joints.

Regarding their bone joints, what is factual—is that the cartilage in the joints has deteriorated: in some cases to where the bone may rub against bone. In addition some joints become inflamed and very painful: affecting either the fingers; the hips; or knees and in some cases maybe even the spine.

One way of checking this popular conviction is for you to scrimmage through the books on arthritis at Barnes and Noble Book Store. In one particular book the author claimed that the cause of arthritis remains a mystery: even though he could explain in medical terms and in detail what happens inside the joints.

Still another assured the reader that arthritis in some form was almost inevitable. That the pain could be taken care of, up to a point, but thereafter not too much could be done.

Some magazines, devoted to health topics, also carried similar dismal news. With some of their contributing authors suggesting a variety of herbal solutions for the pain and discomfort: as an alternative to the normal prescription drugs.

A short while ago our neighbor had a minor fall and broke her wrist. We drove her to a bone specialist and while she was having her wrist put in a cast, we thumbed through some of the magazines in the reception waiting area. Paging through a magazine devoted solely to arthritis it was amazing to learn that the focus of each and every article was to discuss some or other pain relief type medication for arthritics—nowhere was there a mention of a cure or how to avoid getting it in the first place! Nor was there a single mention of any research being done to establish the cause of the deterioration of the cartilage in the first place.

Along the way we seem to have lost the foresight and wisdom of such intelligent people as Thomas Edison. The following quote attributed to him, can be found in Mark Sisson's book *The Primal Blueprint* (ref.6 p.v). We mention Mark since, to be fair, that is where we first saw the quote:

> The doctor of the future will give no medicine,
> but instead will interest his patients in the care
> of human frame, in diet, and in the cause and
> prevention of disease.
>
> Thomas Edison

Sadly it may well be because medicine, in a broader sense and relating to arthritis, seems to have lost the will to establish the cause that Edison's prediction has not yet in the main come to fruition?

If, as one must assume from what is seen around us, that *'not knowing the cause'* is the general situation—it explains the great number of sufferers so afflicted with arthritis. This scary scenario is made worse by the fact we are told the estimated projected rate of increase of the illness, is such it portends an avalanche of suffering—headed toward humanity.

It also adds weight to the argument there is a necessity to remind people of the brilliant work; and the discoveries which can alleviate and eradicate this potential misery—that there is a real urgency to *"rediscover"* what seems to have been so overlooked and forgotten. Consequently, the objective of this book is to bring these positive developments to the fore: and so they are set out in the chapters that follow. The bottom line is there is a need to return to the natural law that states:

> *Nothing just happens—there*
> *has to be a cause or causes!*

What Caused It
—Chapter 3

The sweetest flesh is near the bones.
                                    German Proverb

The above German Proverb was found on Wikiquote.org. (ref.12) It reads in as much as that, "One must attack the root cause; don't try to cure the symptoms—*cure the disease.*"

B.L. was a young engineer employed on research projects in the sugar industry. On one occasion a colleague informed him he had developed a migraine headache, to which B.L. instantly enquired, "What do you think caused it?" From all accounts the colleague was visibly taken aback—as if he had never been asked that sort of question before.

Whoever tries to establish the cause?

Even to where the sufferer is involved. He gets a headache and reaches for the painkillers without a thought as to what brought it on.

Visit any medical doctor and there too it seems the custom is to come away with a script in your hand: always prescribing some medication to treat the symptom. Maybe the poor doctor is in a spot because *patient pressure* dictates this is what is expected in our society today—*give me something to make me well!*

The following personal story was told by Matt in the book, *Help, Thank You!* (ref.22 p.23) His story is titled *Released From Bondage* as it recounts how he suffered with severe migraine headaches for 14 years; before being released from that suffering:

"His headaches started soon after his marriage, becoming worse in intensity and frequency through the years. On some occasions they were so bad his wife needed to ask the doctor to call to their home to give him a sedative so he could sleep through the night.

Doctors' bills and the cost of pain killers and medications weighed on his family. On one occasion a doctor prescribed tranquilizers telling him he was getting the headaches because he could not handle stress. Eventually he settled into a routine of always having a supply of strong painkillers on hand.

Then after about 14 years he and his family took a vacation in the mountains. While there his wife chanced upon a magazine article which claimed that one of the things that caused migraine headaches, was the preservatives being added to foods and candy. The type that was singled out particularly in the article was called *tartrazine.*

The next stage was easy—having chanced upon the *cause,* all he had to do was merely avoid those foods, soups, deserts and candy that contained it. It was that simple: he eliminated the preservatives from his diet—and after 14 years of bondage the headaches disappeared!"

As an aside: if you are ever troubled by recurring headaches or migraine—each time you get one make a note of what you have eaten or drank in the previous 24 to 48 hours. Eventually you will identify the culprit.

Returning to our topic—we know that if your body is invaded by a virus, bacteria or germs then you can become ill. But usually in many cases medicine already knows the cause, through the research done by people like Louis Pasteur and other dedicated chemists and researchers.

However, in the case of arthritis, it has been established microbes or germs are not responsible, and neither is it contagious.

Therefore, one must ask with even more persistence, *"What possibly causes it?"*

And if you are presently arthritis free—then how do you maintain your health and happiness: what is it you must do to avoid developing the symptoms?

Then too, why are some people without the ailment, while so many others have it?

Why do some people reach an old age without contracting arthritis?

Why, when two people live together in the same house—why is it one can get arthritis and the other does not? What is the possible explanation?

And why is it that the incidence of the disease is increasing so rapidly—*almost exponentially?*

Now if arthritis sufferers can find the answers to these questions (and they are available) then the solution is almost as simple as Matt above, finding the cause of his headaches!

In addition there is more good news in that the human body is designed as a self-healing mechanism. You break a leg, and once it is put into splints the bones heal and knit and become repaired: or if you bruise yourself, the body works to heal the damage: or if you tear a ligament or muscle, the body immediately begins healing the tear. The liver for example can even regenerate itself under the right conditions.

So be encouraged by the fact that although you may be in sore straights right now from years of abuse—you can be healed! The only thing that cannot be done is for the deformity to areas of the body such as the fingers and hands to be eradicated. But from what we have seen and read; the inflammation and the pain can be eliminated. Healing shows the rest of the body is once again functioning normally; busily repairing itself.

An excellent book, with the purpose of illustrating how perfectly and beautifully the human body has been made and constructed, is Og Mandino's *The Greatest Miracle in the World* (ref. 13 pp. 93-98). Og Mandino is one of the all time greats at writing self-help books. His description is written in layman terms in the form of a memorandum.

Where Did My Health Go
—Chapter 4

**You don't miss the water
until the well runs dry.**

Irish Proverb

The above was a favorite quote from Don, who is mentioned in the Introduction. He would use it whenever it was appropriate to caution a family member or friend to take care of, and treasure one's health while they still possessed it. His motto was, "Do not wait until you have a heart attack before you modify your lifestyle." Another equally appropriate quote of his was:

"No one repairs the leak in the
roof while the sun shines."

H.F. was a medical doctor. When he went for an annual checkup with a colleague it was discovered certain arteries had a very high blockage due to the presence of bad fats or bad cholesterol in the veins. Before his examination he had not been too concerned with what he ate: but after his procedure to clear the arteries he became very diet conscious—making time to read the nutrition and health books. He became intent on discovering what mistakes he had made to cause the problem.

The great tragedy is that in spite of the knowledge and education of people today; and the sophistication of society in general—we seem to be like the early Romans: so sure we have it made, but with the nation as a whole committing an obvious blunder. And no one—except the enlightened people we are about to quote—are asking, "Why is this happening to society en masse?

Surely, someone should be comparing what society is doing today with what it did when people were generally a lot healthier. The statistics relating to obesity, diabetes, arthritis and heart attacks should be prompting those sorts of questions. Dr. Richard J. Johnson (ref.8 p.3 and p.11) has said that a century ago, few Americans were overweight with relatively low rates of diabetes – but that today diabetes affects more than 20 million Americans. His statistics concerning high blood pressure shows it has increased by 20 per cent over the past 30 years and now affects about 73 million people.

Wikipedia (ref.10) has this disturbing report concerning children:

"Traditionally considered a disease of adults, type-2 diabetes is increasingly diagnosed in children in parallel with rising obesity rates."

On Wednesday July 10, 2013, all major TV stations, reported on the recent findings of the United Nations—that Mexico had now overtaken the USA in obesity rates amongst its peoples. The report stated that nearly 70 percent of Mexican adults are overweight and that childhood obesity in the country had tripled within the past decade.

Particularly disturbing was the scenario that nearly 70,000 deaths in Mexico each year are caused by weight-related diabetes, and more than 400,000 new cases of diabetes are diagnosed annually.

Sadly we did not hear of any planned or pending investigation to discover the root cause of this problem in what is now clearly becoming an epidemic.

It is important to note that the increases in these maladies have occurred in the recent 50 to 75 years—because highlighting this fact ties in with the increases of the factors causing the problem: or that which people as a whole are doing wrong!

More resolute than ever, we continue with our own investigation and ask this question:

Where Did My Health Go?

Where did my health go?
For lack of it is beginning to show.

Once I walked tall and straight;
Now, I walk with a stoop of late.

Other people dance and play;
When I leave they want me to stay.

Once I had boundless energy;
Now, I just want to be let be.

These knees of mine squeak and creak.
When people hear I feel a right geek.

My fingers are all bent and skew;
How I wish they could be made like new.

In a motorized cart I am a prize goof;
The thought of it drives me through the roof.

Doctors and druggists keep sending me bills;
Why should I fill cash register tills?

An apple a day did keep those away;
Now there's nothing to hold them at bay.

Where did my health go?
I would so like to know.

We are blessed in that there are answers to that plea; which have been put forward by brilliant researchers. Answers which have been tried and tested: and proved correct. The bottom line is—*if you know what causes it you can "fix it" and restore your health and happiness.*

Some people think there is no cure?
But there is, of this I know for sure.

Ending in a wheelchair does not have to be;
For knowledge of the causes will set you free.

However, a good way to begin—to ensure the thinking of these distinguished researchers is appreciated and understood—is with one of the medical giants from history.

Louis Pasteur
—Chapter 5

Cleanliness is next to Godliness
Ancient Hebrew Proverb

An easy and enjoyable way to get to know about this man, his theories, his work and his achievements is to view the movie *Louis Pasteur,* starring Paul Muni in the main role. Although the movie (ref.23) was made in 1936, and is in black and white—it is very enjoyable and very informative.

His active working years were during the period childbirth was to be feared by women. Statistics, from those times, show three out of 10 mothers died soon after giving birth. Of course, we all now know it was from disease contracted because of lack of sterilization of instruments used in midwifery—and in particular because doctors did not deem it necessary to wash their hands before assisting with a delivery.

However, you are encouraged to watch the movie, or read a book on Pasteur, because the attitude of the medical profession, in certain scenarios, has not changed much since that time. And in those areas; just as before when they thought they knew it all—there seems a majority who scoff at any suggestion they could possibly be in the wrong.

Should you be unable to view the movie, here is a brief description:

The movie starts by depicting the year 1860: with Pasteur distributing pamphlets advising the citizens of Paris to insist their doctors—*Wash their hands and boil their instruments: that microbes cause disease and death to their patients.*

He is then ostracized and subjected to ridicule by the eminent physicians and doctors of his day. He is considered a quack, a charlatan and mountebank within the medical community. He is after that almost totally isolated from the doctors of his time.

Although he did not practice medicine—he was a chemist—he tries to put a stop to the negligence of those who were. Probably because he was a chemist is what enabled him to discover the germs that transmitted disease. The premise of the important professional physicians at the time, on the other hand, is how could a small organism such as a microbe affect or harm our large bodies.

The animosity towards him grows to such an extent he is virtually forced to leave Paris and retires to the country. Fortunately for mankind, while there he sets up his laboratory again and tackles the problems affecting farmers in his vicinity.

After the Franco-Prussian war in 1870, the French government notices that in the area where Pasteur resides the incidence of anthrax—endemic in the rest of France—is virtually non-existent.

It turns out this is because he has successfully developed a vaccine which has eliminated the disease from the local farm animals.

His vaccine is *put to the test* and we get to see how it is proved to be successful—raising the livestock output of France.

His dedication and hard work increase and—in spite of the continued resistance and opposition from the medical experts—he proceeds to develop a vaccine for hydrophobia or rabies. His passion to save people unnecessary death from this infection is evidenced in the movie.

Towards the end of the movie his theories regarding germs are accepted, and he is singularly awarded by the medical council in Paris: with a general acclaim for his achievements. While addressing the young doctors and scientists at the ceremony he encourages them to always work towards contributing in some way to the welfare of mankind. His closing remark is they should take heart because:

> **No scientific theory has ever been
> accepted without opposition.**
>
> Louis Pasteur

While researching Louis Pasteur and his theories, a research paper was chanced upon. It is written by Professor Christine L. Case and titled *Hand Washing* (ref. 15). Of particular interest in her article is how opponents of hygiene existed in the early 20th century.

In her excellent article Professor Case tells how in 1910 a Dr. Josephine Baker began teaching hygiene to child care providers in New York. Later, as a consequence of the success Dr. Baker was achieving; 30 physicians sent a petition to the Mayor protesting that *it was ruining medical practice by...keeping babies well.*

Later on, in her article, we were surprised to read that even today "hand washing is insufficiently practiced as a means of inhibiting the spread of infectious germs."

Professor Case goes on to cite the case that in 1993; 11 healthcare workers all became ill with hepatitis A; because they did not wash their hands after treating a patient with hepatitis A.

Her article is good and worth a read as there is much of value in it.

Something else that is so amazing is the more elaborate and risky and expensive the treatment: the more folk are enamored with it.

A short time ago, a woman, E.B. told about the medication she was taking for her arthritis. E.B. said it was so potentially harmful to her stomach that she could only take it at mealtimes. In addition, as a precaution, she had to take another medication a half hour before mealtimes: to ensure there would be no reaction from the potent medication she was to take with her meal.

There comes a time surely, for those on regular prescription medications, to sit back and ask, "All these pain killers and such—what are they doing to my important body organs such as my intestines, liver and kidneys?"

Be careful—*protect yourself!*

Profit Motive In Selling
—Chapter 6

A burnt child dreads the fire.
English Proverb

E.W. was a chief engineer in charge of the maintenance and production departments in a manufacturing concern. At one particular meeting he addressed his senior staff regarding the advertisements they had to peruse when looking for equipment. He said, "Be on your guard when there is a beautiful and scantily dressed model posing with the equipment. They are attempting to distract you—so you do not see the flaws in what they are selling!"

P.T. was a young teenager, still at school. He was an avid listener of the radio, and had become enchanted with a particular advertisement that included a very "catchy" tune; so much so he would often hum it. Now this particular advert promised health and happiness throughout the day—if you took their brand of fruit-salts (an antacid) each morning.

Telling his story, P.T. said he had begged his parents to buy the product so he could take it: which they did. But then suddenly he was blessed through an unfortunate event involving his father, who had become ill and was hospitalized. While there he was placed in a general ward, and in the bed alongside of him there had been a 21 year old youth.

This particular young man had become so addicted to the very same antacid which P.T. had bought—that his body could no longer *operate* without it. The whole reason for hospitalizing him had been to wean him off the antacid in a controlled medical environment.

P.T. said for his father to have encountered the youth in a hospital—so he himself could be warned of the danger of taking the antacid; was an act of Providence. It was his first awakening experience to the fact that a manufacturer could sell a product, even though it was harmful to the consumer, as a means to making money.

It is pertinent to point out here that folk can develop an *acid stomach* when they overindulge in wrong foods such as cakes, pastries, etc. Taking an antacid gives the impression of it being beneficial because the *acid feeling* disappears. This happens because the hydrochloric acid in the stomach gets neutralized!

If the person then eats protein he is *in trouble!* To digest it he needs hydrochloric acid—but the acid has been *used up* so to speak by the neutralizing action of the antacid. Consequently the pancreas has to work overtime. One should note this is what happens each time an antacid is taken. Taking it regularly places an enormous load on the pancreas that wears it out over time.

Far better to give up the bad foods causing the acidity in the first place!

J.W. was a young man in his early twenties. He mentioned that in the large coastal city, where he grew up, was a huge shipping terminal used exclusively for loading cargo vessels with export sugar. On the terminal towers was a prominent sign, which was visible for miles around, with a very clever drawing of a teaspoon carrying a load of sugar: and below it was the slogan, *"Sugar gives you go."*

He said he believed it: possibly, because it justified his craving for chocolate. But nonetheless it was effective advertising because it confirmed his belief that eating sugar would increase his energy levels: thus he justified his chocolate expenses.

J.W. also told of another advert from his younger years in the form of a jingle over the radio—from the makers of Cadburys. It went, *"There's a glass and a half of fresh cream milk in Cadburys—Cadburys Dairy Milk chocolate."* He said it was so effective, he truly assumed that in eating their chocolate, he was eating nutrition!

It has been said that advertizing is mostly directed at people below the age of 40—because by that age folk are set in their ways: or have come to realize that advertizing is a serious business. It costs a lot to advertize, especially on TV. Therefore the whole object of advertizing is to get you to buy the product—the more you buy the greater the success of the campaign—with the object being to recoup the costs many times over: and to increase producer sales. It is all about *money being the name of the game.* Your welfare is way down on the chart.

B.H. told of the time he was in high school, and was celebrating a friend's birthday with him along with his classmates. The friend's father worked as a manager in a bakery, and had sent them cream cakes and pastries for the occasion. They were so delicious that BH said he was sure fresh cream had been used. Anyhow, because they were 'mouth-watering' delicious, he asked how the cream had been made.

The birthday lad was able to answer the question because, as it turned out, his father had taken him many times to the bakery, making the cakes: so he knew firsthand how the cream had been made. B.H. remembers he was flabbergasted when informed the cream was an imitation—made solely from the cheap ingredients of lard (rendered animal fat) mixed with confectioners powdered sugar. It had been blended so well it tasted like fresh cream. But it was a most useful learning experience. It taught him how manufacturers are able to reduce costs and simultaneously increase the shelf-life—in this case by using mock ingredients rather than natural cream.

S.Q. was the proprietor of a manufacturing concern. On one occasion the owner of a neighboring factory, who made orange juice, came to visit. This fellow packaged his orange juice product in small convenient size plastic bottles for sale to people on their way to work in the morning.

He shared with S.Q. how he had reduced his input costs to the minimum by substituting with artificial orange juice ingredients, and artificial sweeteners. However he was upset since he could not totally use the artificial sweeteners, because if he did the 'juice' turned black. The most he could use was 50 percent—the other half being made up of sugar or sucrose: which was more expensive than the sweetener.

Consequently, in this case scenario, there were people on their way to work in the morning thinking they were buying real orange juice—but what they were purchasing was a concoction of chemicals. Good for profits though!

In his excellent book *The Sugar Fix* Dr. Richard J. Johnson (ref.21 p.27) tells how in November 1984, the makers of Coca-Cola and Pepsi decided to replace refined sugar with high-fructose corn syrup (HFCS) in the USA, to reduce the cost of sweeteners in their soft drinks.

What has all this to do with the arthritic?

It is extremely important for one to be aware that corporations exist to make profits—the greater the money made—the more their objectives are met. In the USA the drug industry generates billions and billions. It is a great business: and the proportion coming from arthritic patients is huge. A few years ago there was a newspaper article telling how some doctors actually receive bonuses, from pharmaceutical companies; depending upon the amount of drugs they prescribed to patients.

So you need to *keep an eye out* when seeking services or medications. Unfortunately, there are some people who will willingly, 'take that dollar out of your pocket and put it into theirs.'

Consequently, also keep an open mind when reviewing advice offered in commercials through media, newspapers, and such. Always ask the question, *"What are they trying to sell me? What's in it for them? Will they profit at my expense? Is there not perhaps a better way for me—a way that is more beneficial to my overall health?"*

The Road To Discovery
—Chapter 7

"As I see it, every day you
do one of two things:
build health or produce
disease in yourself."
Adelle Davis

Unwittingly, my wife and I had been producing disease in ourselves—and it was becoming clearly visible in the early symptoms of arthritis: as recounted in the Foreword.

To be brief, we had relocated to a new continent with a much colder climate than we were formerly accustomed. To remain healthy and avoid catching colds or influenza, we had agreed to have grapefruit at breakfast: and then to eat several oranges during the day—for the vitamin C. In addition we had a super recipe for roasting fresh raw peanuts, and snacked on these several times during the day as well. Then, as a *cheer-me-up* we made homemade fudge, which was eaten frequently.

After our meeting with Peggy, we purchased Dale Alexander's *Arthritis and Common Sense* (ref. 2) and began reading it immediately—from cover to cover.

To our surprise we discovered that all the above things we were eating—the grapefruit, the oranges, the peanuts and the fudge—were contributing to the onset of the arthritis!

According to Alexander it seemed the sugar in the fudge was the number one culprit. After that it was the grapefruit, because of its acidic nature, and then the oranges. The peanuts did not escape blame either, as they too were doing their share of damage.

Regarding the peanuts—these we eliminated from the diet largely because Alexander recommended we do so. Other than say they contained the wrong type of oils; he gave no further supporting reasons for why we should abstain. Neither did he specify exactly what he meant by *wrong oils* and it is only now; while reading the latest research, that we understand peanuts are very high in omega-6 oils or fatty acids. And if eaten in quantity create an imbalance in the diet with the omega-3 oils, or fatty acids. Generally, the Western diet is already largely deficient in omega-3 (as was ours at the time): consequently by eating foods high in omega-6; and not eating foods with omega-3, we were making the imbalance worse—which was seriously harming our health.

Incidentally, all the foods mainly recommended by Alexander for arthritics contain omega-3 oils, although in varying amounts.

What helped make Alexander's theories believable was our earlier introduction to *Body Mind & Sugar* by E.M. Abrahamson,

M.D and A.W. Pezet (ref. 3). Dr. Abrahamson had convincingly warned strongly of the dangers of including sugar in the diet. His compelling explanations of the harm being done to the body; made it easier for us to accept as true what Alexander was saying.

To make a long story short, by following Alexander's recommendations—switching to eating the healthy foods he suggested along with taking cod liver oil in the manner he prescribed —we began to heal: and within a period of six months our arthritic symptoms had disappeared.

On the subject of preferred medications for arthritis—the only thing Alexander really recommends is taking cod liver oil. It is his panacea or cure-all. But a word of caution: the cod liver oil today is far more concentrated—in terms of the quantity of vitamin A and D—than it was when he wrote his book. Therefore, it should not be taken in the quantities he recommended at that time. (Please note that the dosage for cod liver oil is later discussed in Chapter 14 *Essential Oils.*)

Our experience with arthritis occurred over 15 years ago and to this day my wife has remained arthritis free. As for me I did not take one of the other causes given by Alexander seriously enough and the ailment returned slightly about a year ago. In a way this is fortunate as I now have additional experience regarding his theories and can say, "He knew what he was talking about." This latest excursion into "producing disease within me" is discussed later in Chapter 12, *Another Cause of Arthritis.*

The Foreword in Alexander's book (ref.2 p.1) was written by Doctor H. E. Kirschner who personally testifies how he witnessed two people being cured through Alexander's methods.

The first occasion he describes is how a former patient was cured, when she took the lubricating oils. Doctor Kirschner says it was a miracle to see how she improved.

The other healing incident he describes was when a 10 year old child, who had been afflicted with rheumatoid arthritis, was cured. He said for five years she had been given every type of medical treatment—but that she only responded when her diet was corrected and given cod liver oil.

Wanting to know more about Doctor Kirschner we did a search on Google and there discovered he had done sterling work in healing other patients, from different diseases, through administering cod liver oil; and in particular by using juicing.

Returning to Alexander's book, the statistics he offers are in line with other researchers and doctors, who say that at age 60 there is a 60 percent probability the average person will have arthritis in some degree of severity. Those figures remind one of the early Romans who had a 66 percent chance of developing gout in their later years—a form of arthritis—albeit from a different cause. (We cannot help but wonder if historians of the future will one day maybe compare our civilization with that of the Romans?) In general, arthritis seems to affect men firstly in the knees—while in women the joints that are affected first, are in the fingers and hands; then the knees: and for both groups the hips and spine are likely to follow.

However, before evaluating the substance which is *the #1 Cause of Arthritis,* in the next Chapter, it is necessary to understand why its harmful effects are not more readily recognized by folk and doctors in general.

Essentially it is because basically the human body is its own worst enemy!

How is this?

It is because the body has been designed as the most efficient self-healing entity.

You scratch yourself and it heals. You break a leg and after it is splinted and set, the bones knit and join together again. Get a bruise from a bump, or kick, and in time it disappears as the body silently works at healing the cells.

It even compensates for the wrong or spoilt foods you may eat: more so than with animals or creatures. Because we have a more varied diet than animals the body can take nutrients from the good foods to process the bad foods, to an extent.

M.N. was a young man who lived in a city that boasted a crocodile farm as a tourist attraction. Then one day he read an account in the local newspaper that a nutritionist had been called in because the baby crocodiles were becoming deformed a few weeks after hatching.

A follow up article, a few weeks later, reported that the cause of the problem had been established. The diet being fed the baby crocodiles lacked certain nutrients—and as soon as the diet was altered the crocodiles grew normally. Because their diet happened to be so restricted, with virtually one item on the menu so to speak; it was easy to establish the cause of the deformities.

But it is not so easy with humans.

People, on the other hand, eat a cross section of all types of food. In one way it is a saving grace—but the downside is that the harmful effects of some foods and substances can remain undetected for very long periods.

Consider the case of a person who happens to eat rancid peanuts. The body then has to process them and expel the harmful substances and poisons they contain. However, to do so *it uses up* the good nutrients and vitamins in the body, or that is in the other good food being eaten: or both. This in turn robs the body of the essential *goodness* needed to function and remain healthy.

As example, if one has a diet consisting largely of healthy vegetables and protein foods the problem of eating stuff that is bad for you can remain hidden for many years—often into old age. But it eventually catches up with you because there is only so much the poor old body can do; without the proper resources and nutrients.

Further, the reason we have this high incidence and prevalence of arthritis, diabetes, cancers and cardiac arrests, etc. in our society today—is because, *the harmful substances part of our diet,* is increasing while the good stuff with the nutrients and vitamins is being discarded.

For that reason, be thankful if your body is "notifying you things are not right" with a minor ailment like the early stages of arthritis. By alerting you there is a problem; you can take the necessary action to restore your health.

Encouragingly, if your condition is more advanced—you too will be amazed at how your body's healing mechanism will respond if you create the right conditions. Be filled with hope because your can heal, as Dr. Bass has said:

The recuperative power of the human
body from illness to health can only
be described as little short of amazing.

Dr. Bass

Listen carefully to the arguments below. These arise from
the dedicated work of eminent researchers and doctors who have
studied the effects of these substances on ailments like arthritis
and other diseases. Then seek out and evaluate *the evidence that is
all around you:* as suggested in Chapter 9 below.

The #1 Cause Of Arthritis
—Chapter 8

**It is a travesty that a substance
which is so bad for you,
can taste so good.**

This chapter consists of three sections:

- How the body "burns" glucose
- The make-up of sugars, and
- Reports from medical doctors and researchers

How the body "burns" glucose

The way I see it, you must *'burn'* fuel to obtain the energy in it.

An example is the engine in your motor vehicle, and how it is designed to *'burn'* gasoline. As the gasoline ignites it turns into gas, expands and the energy thus derived is used to move the pistons, so turning the gear train and eventually the wheels. For the engine to burn the gasoline oxygen is required. The oxygen enters the piston chamber as part of the air that is drawn into the engine along with the gasoline.

In burning this fuel heat is given off, to such an extent a cooling system must be attached to the motor so it will cool, and remain at running temperature.

Similarly, another fuel such as coal can be burnt in a controlled environment, as in a furnace, from where the heat can be used, say, to turn water into steam. One use for the steam is to drive generators and so generate electricity. Once more, oxygen is needed and this is obtained from the air supply flowing over the fuel.

You can easily test this claim that a fire *breathes* in as much as it requires oxygen to burn fuel. Simply stand a candle with a large base (so it will not fall over) in a plate and obtain a glass jar large enough that when it is upended it will cover the candle and leave a space between the flame and the base of the jar. Next pour a small amount of water in the plate to form a seal with the upended jar. When you are set up; light the candle and place the jar over it. It will burn brightly until the oxygen in the air in the jar is used up—then it sputters and goes out.

Now for your body to get energy it also must *burn fuel*. You require this energy so your muscles can operate for you to walk, or move around in general. Organs inside your body, such as the heart, lungs, stomach, brain, etc. need a constant supply of energy so they will operate in the way they were designed.

And in the same way that your car engine gets hot—so too does your body when it burns fuel to work hard: as when you run or do strenuous exercise. It even has a 'built-in' cooling system. You get hot and then perspire. The latent heat required to turn the perspiration into vapor is taken from the surface of the body—and so you are cooled.

However, the marked difference is you cannot have a 'fire' in your body, obviously!

Therefore, the body is designed to *burn fuel* through a series of chemical reactions. Any foods you eat, be it carbohydrates, sugars, fruits or even protein—that are to be used as fuel by the body—are eventually turned into glucose through a series of chemical reactions.

To simplify our explanation, we will go straight to the final chemical reaction, which is the *burning* of the glucose—and is actually the reaction between the glucose and the insulin.

The glucose can come via the stomach walls, intestines or from the liver—depending on what kind of sugars have been eaten and at what stage the sugar absorption or storage process is at. The blood carries it to where it is needed.

Insulin is manufactured in the pancreas and taken by the blood to where in the body it is needed. This *burning of glucose* is what gives the energy. However, as with any *fire* there has to be oxygen which is brought from the lungs after being extracted from the air one breathes.

But where the body is concerned there is an extra requirement in the burning process because of the series of chemical reactions—and this is so important to understand—*that for any chemical reaction to take place there has to be a catalyst.*

Without a catalyst, a chemical reaction cannot occur. The catalyst does not become part of the compound—it gets "used up so to speak" while aiding and making it possible for the reaction to take place.

Now the catalyst required in the body—for the reaction between the glucose and the insulin to occur—is in effect the essential nutrients and vitamins, found in foods, i.e. vitamin C and some of the B vitamins; along with others.

Even the humble potato contains vitamin C, plus other vitamins, to enable the body to utilize the carbohydrate. This explains why there are large quantities of vitamin C in those sugar containing foods we eat. The higher the fructose or sugar: the greater concentrations of vitamin C.

In a healthy person insulin is made and released into the bloodstream as and when the body needs it to process the sugar and carbohydrate. To obtain a deeper insight read the excellent resume of how insulin is produced in the pancreas—in fact in glands called 'the islands of langerans'—which is given in Dr. Abrahamson's book *Body, Mind and Sugar* (ref.3).

For use in-between meals your body *stores excess sugar*, or glucose, in the liver as glycogen. When it is required, the liver releases the glycogen which is then converted back to glucose and carried by the blood stream to where it is needed.

Importantly, your body is *run and managed* by your subconscious as if it is on *"autopilot."* It does this in a way you are not even aware of the multiplicity of different decisions and actions that are being constantly made to ensure its smooth operation inside of you—while both awake and asleep. Even when it is in "crisis mode" of operation you may not be aware—it is only if the situation worsens, say you feel faint or ill—you become aware it is in trouble.

As you consume different foods the "sensors" in the body's digestive tract detect them and the sub-conscious "decides" what enzymes, along with acid, to release and how much. This is by and large a relatively *slow process* if you eat normal slow digesting healthy foods. In any event, as the foods eaten are digested the monitoring continues—and as new foods, or needs, are detected the pancreas and stomach adjust accordingly. It can take up to three hours for the stomach to digest a regular meal, and for a protein steak dinner it can take up to four hours. Further digestion is continued in the intestines.

Before the advent of refined sugar and white flour; man obtained his sugars as a result of eating fruits, whole cereals and other slow digesting foods: giving the digestive process time to act in a slow and well orchestrated manner. Very importantly, this meant carbohydrates and sugars were ingested slowly. The body had plenty of time to go through the different chemical reaction processes and finally convert them into glucose for immediate energy; or to store the glucose as glycogen—or body fat if the glycogen reserves were "full."

But with the advent of modern machinery: man began refining his foods. This has occurred extensively during the last 200 years—and in the last 50 years: *the use of refined foods has and is increasing almost exponentially.*

The thing about refined foods such as sugar or sucrose and white flour is they can be converted almost instantly into glucose. In fact pure sugar crystals are roughly 50 percent glucose and 50 percent fructose. What that in essence means is that the glucose part of the sugar is absorbed immediately through the stomach walls and into the blood stream:

That is as good as to being given an injection
of pure glucose directly into an artery or vein!

In his brilliant book Dr. Abrahamson (ref.3 p.36) states that there is the equivalent of two teaspoons of blood sugars, or rather glucose, in the blood stream of a healthy person at any given time. If these sugars fall below that level the body works to restore them by utilizing the reserves of glycogen. If the level of glucose rises above two teaspoons the body immediately begins converting the excess into glycogen, or body fats.

The *"sub-conscious knows"* that if the glucose levels fall too far the body is in trouble—the brain and heart can be affected. If the levels rise too high the individual could lapse into a diabetic coma, or experience blindness. In the extreme he could die! The controlling mechanism in the body is totally aware of this state of affairs.

It is important to restate that:

There are two teaspoons of glucose in
the blood stream at any one time!

Very roughly, two teaspoons equals about 12gm in weight.

Now along comes pure unadulterated sugar—pure crystals that are devoid of the vitamins and minerals necessary for *the burning or combustion,* in the chemical reaction processes.

Consider this scenario.

You 'down' a 12oz coke—that contains 39gm of sugar; that is approximately 6½ teaspoons—which is in the form of fructose. This fructose is speedily and rapidly assimilated through the stomach and intestines. You are totally unaware of it—*but the "air raid sirens" are being set off in your subconscious:*

And the message is, "We are under attack!"

This finely designed body of yours goes into preservation mode—it has been invaded by 6½ teaspoons of a lethal substance *(lethal in the sense that if this sugar invading the system is allowed to exceed the two teaspoons—then coma or even death can result).*

So the communication goes out, "Secrete insulin rapidly to convert this excess sugar into glycogen for storage in the liver." Your body's response may even be to secrete adrenalin—the fight or flight drug—to get the system to operate more promptly and efficiently, converting this excess glucose. The message is clear:

This battle has to, must be won at all costs.

By *pulling out all the stops* the pancreas rapidly makes and secrets insulin and so the particular battle is won. *But at a price!* The problem is that over many years of having to produce at such a rapid basis causes the islands of langerans to lose their sensitivity—and eventually in the haste to be effective, they start over-producing. Too much insulin not only *uses up* the sugar consumed; but it now starts to *use up* the sugar that was free flowing in your blood—and the levels fall below the required two teaspoons.

This results in another emergency message to release glycogen from the liver—with the consequent whipsaw action as your body tries to maintain stability. And as Dr. Abrahamson points out this eventually leads to hypoglycemia or hyperinsulinism—where the individual begins to suffer from low blood sugars.

In the case of the diabetic the islands of langerans get so worn out they lose the ability to make insulin.

The problems are magnified if the person drinks several sodas during the day and also eats chocolates and desserts all containing sugars.

Because of the refining process the scenario of the man 'downing' a coke, or eating a slab of chocolate, is made much worse because the *sugars are devoid of vitamins and nutrients*—the catalysts necessary for the chemical reaction processes to achieve the combustion of the glucose.

But the reaction has to take place to get rid of this excess sugar—or you die!

So what does the body in trouble do? It seeks out those vitamins and nutrients necessary to process the sugars from other foods being consumed. If the individual has eaten plenty of vegetables containing the necessary vitamins and nutrients he may be okay in the short term. (Longer term, there are other serious hazards from the sugar intake.) But if the meal largely consists of refined processed foods, lacking vitamins and nutrients, *then the body is in real danger because the person is now very short of vitamins.*

Accordingly, if it is short on vitamins, the digestive process searches elsewhere—*and it robs your body cells of the vitamins and nutrients that are stored in them.* It must have these to execute the chemical reaction—and that is when, over a period of time and depending on the amount of sugar consumed daily, with this constant depletion of vitamins in the cells, that the *rot literally sets in:* within the body cells.

For the arthritic the excess fructose part of the sugar—forms uric acid and other compounds which travel to the joints, where damage occurs. And while sugar is being absorbed through the intestines; it also does real harm (because of the nature of the substance), in destroying the intestinal walls: making it difficult for what vitamins and minerals there are in the diet, subsequently to be absorbed.

There is further damage because in addition the sugar also destroys the friendly bacteria in the intestines. These friendly gut bacteria are required to help with the digestion of the food; and the manufacture of some B vitamins.

In his book Dr. Abrahamson (ref.3 pp.10-11) gives an important overview of this sugar burning process, based on experience with one of his patients. This particular patient had come to him with a sugar problem. As a means of helping the fellow he originally prescribed glucose tablets that were to be taken each time he experienced a low blood sugar attack.

He describes how his patient bought a box of then and went home. At first they worked fine. Each time he got an attack he took a tablet and recovered. But soon the attacks started occurring more frequently—so much so he started buying the dextrose by the case. Eventually he was unable to sleep through the night without taking the tablets—in due course taking them almost without waking.

Dr. Abrahamson goes on to state that ultimately his patient was eating so much dextrose he was becoming obese. He said his patient's islands of langerans were too sensitive and overgenerous. Instead of making only the amount of insulin needed to handle the amount of sugar just taken into the blood, an excess of insulin was produced, later causing another drop in his blood sugar. His symptoms then returned and with them a demand for more glucose.

A solution arrived when he came across the work of Dr. Seale Harris—professor of medicine at the University of Alabama, who had initially discovered the problems, associated with eating sugar and refined foods; and had then developed special diets to restore health.

The patient was treated according to Dr. Harris' directives and he soon completely recovered.

The make-up of sugars

Sucrose is derived from sugar cane and sugar beet. It is very roughly 50 per cent fructose and 50 percent glucose. Towards the end of the last century a new sugar was produced, viz. high fructose corn syrup (HFCS).

Wikipedia.org (ref. 10) gives these statistics and a fact (emphasis added):

"The world produced about 168 million tonnes of sugar in 2011. The average person consumes about 24 kilograms of sugar each year (33.1 kg in industrialized countries), equivalent to over 260 food calories per person, per day. _Sugar provides energy but no nutrients—{it is considered as} empty calories."_

Sally Fallon with Mary G. Enig, PhD in their book _Nourishing Nutrition_ (ref.11 p.21) say this about refining sugar, and grains (again with emphasis added):

"The refining process strips grains, vegetables and fruits of both their vitamin and mineral components. _"Negative calories" is a better word than "empty calories" because they need your precious reserves to process them."_

We first read about the New Jersey dentist Dr. Robert Boesler, in William Dufty's book _Sugar Blues_ (ref.20 p.42). Then searching on Google we came across other quotes from this brilliant man. Thus he stated in 1912 that, "Modern manufacturing of sugar has brought about entirely new diseases. Sugar has caused a vast degeneration of the people." And that, _"The sugar of commerce is nothing else but concentrated crystallized acid."_

If you Google the makeup of sugar a host of sites appear. TheDailyGreen.com gives this useful overview of the different types of sugars:

Glucose is the sugar in blood, and dextrose is the name given to glucose produced from corn. Biochemically they are identical.

Fructose is the principal sugar in fruit. In fruit, it raises no issues because it is accompanied by nutrients and fiber.

Sucrose is table sugar. It is a double sugar, containing one part each of glucose (50%) and fructose (50%), chemically bound together. Enzymes in the intestine quickly and efficiently split sucrose into glucose and fructose, which are absorbed into the body as single sugars.

HFCS is made from corn starch. It contains roughly equivalent amounts of glucose (45 to 58%) and fructose (42 to 55%).

Reports of medical doctors and researchers

Wikipedia.org (ref. 10) is a favorite site, and regarding degenerative diseases there is this pertinent quote from Dr. Otto H. Warburg:

"Cancer, above all other diseases, has countless secondary causes. But, even for cancer, there is only one prime cause. Summarized in a few words, the prime cause of cancer is the replacement of the respiration of oxygen in normal body cells by a fermentation of sugar."

It will be worth your while to access Wikipedia and read their full page on Dr. Otto Warburg—it is very illuminating. In the meantime the comments on Wikipedia are supported by Sally Fallon in "Nourishing Nutrition" (ref.11 p.24)

"Sugar consumption is positively associated with cancer in humans and test animals. Tumors are known to be enormous sugar absorbers. Sugar is the cause of bone loss and dental decay......Sugar causes tooth decay not because it promotes bacterial growth—but because it alters the internal body chemistry."

An interesting account of sailors being shipwrecked in 1793; is given by William Dufty in his book (ref.20 p.136). He tells how their ship was carrying a cargo of sugar and when the food ran out after being shipwrecked, they began eating the sugar.

When they were rescued, after nine days of eating nothing but sugar and drinking rum, they were in a wasted condition due to starvation. It seems that by only drinking plain water one can stay alive for some time—but sugar robs the body of essential nutrients to process it; causing the excessive wasting.

While we seem to be straying into the field of cancer and other diseases—this overall appreciation of the detrimental effects of sugar must surely help the arthritic to avoid it like the plague.

Something else one needs to be aware of is the harm that can be done through an excessive amount of caffeine. Maybe you should check this out yourself in Dr. Abrahamson's book (ref.3 p.65). He maintains that while overindulgence in sweets (sugar) tends to sensitize the islands of Langerans by subjecting them to repeated stimulation and exercise. Caffeine stimulates the adrenal cortex to produce more of its hormones, which in turn induce the liver to break down glycogen into glucose which flows into the blood stream. Basically, this means the caffeine will cause a rise and fall in your blood sugar levels, with the adverse effects discussed above.

Forewarned, allows you to plan and eat regularly with decent food and so keep your sugar levels elevated. This is why people with hypoglycemia (hyperinsulinism) eat small meals frequently.

Very fortunately, we subsequently also stumbled upon the more recent book from Dr. Richard J. Johnson titled *The Sugar Fix* (ref.8). In it he illustrates the detrimental effect to your health from high fructose corn syrup (HFCS). He shows from his scientific studies and research exactly the harm that comes from consuming too much of this fructose. He also warns that the harmful sucrose (sugar) we have been discussing is 50 percent fructose.

Dr. Johnson (ref.8 p.7) states that, from his research, there is mounting scientific evidence that consuming too much fructose makes one fat and increases the risk for high blood pressure, heart disease; diabetes and kidney disease. This is because (ref.8 p.14), a high fructose diet raises levels of *unhealthy blood fats* and lowers your good cholesterol levels.

Dr. Johnson further states that a high intake of fructose stimulates the production of uric acid. *And that uric acid has an adverse effect on blood pressure.* This is tremendously important to be aware of if you want to maintain your health.

He has opened new boundaries regarding sugars in the diet by highlighting the ill effects of fructose. HFCS, especially in sodas and fruit juices, is rapidly absorbed into the blood stream where it immediately upsets the sugar balance. But surprisingly, fructose is also available in fruits. Consequently, if you have a sugar problem you will want to limit your fruit intake: and when eating fruit do so after a meal where it can be processed slowly with the other food eaten.

Dr. Joseph Mercola (ref.17) has his own health site, viz. Mercola.com. He has this to say regarding sugar in his posting on 5/7/13:

"Avoid Sugar and Processed Foods. Sugar impairs the quality of your immune response almost immediately, and as you likely know, a healthy immune system is one of the most important keys to fighting off viruses and other illness.

It also can decimate your beneficial bacteria and feed the pathogenic yeast and viruses. Be aware that sugar (typically in the form of high fructose corn syrup) is present in foods you may not suspect, like ketchup and fruit juice."

The eminent cardiologist Dr. William Davis, in his book *Wheat Belly* (ref.9 p.33) has done sterling work in highlighting the dangers of highly refined, highly processed and genetically modified foods—his main theme being the harm modern wheat, can do to you. He says that whole wheat bread available today in reality increases blood sugar to a higher level than sucrose. In fact he goes onto say that two slices of whole wheat bread can be worse than drinking a can of sugar-sweetened soda.

His book is really informative as one discovers that the wheat grown nowadays has been so modified it no longer has the same nutritional value as that which children were fed 50 years ago. What is so bad about the wheat these days is that the body rapidly converts it to fat.

You can verify for yourself that what he says is true. Eat three or four slices of bread during the day—then jump on your scale next morning!

Dr. Davis has good news for arthritics—he verifies that arthritis can be cured, as can diabetes. You will need to read his full report (ref.9 p.9), concerning his patients. But he clearly states that only after three months of having been taken off refined carbohydrates—sugar and wheat, etc. their blood sugar levels had dropped from the diabetic range to normal. Meaning his diabetics become *non*-diabetics!

Regarding his arthritic patients he noted that by removing carbohydrates, especially wheat, from the diet their rheumatoid arthritis pain improved or disappeared completely. This enabled them to cut back, or even to eliminate, the medications they were using.

Importantly for us, Dr. Davis (ref.9 p.125) verifies Alexander's original work with his own research when he says it is the high blood sugars—an excess amount of sugar in the blood from eating the rapidly absorbable sucrose or sugar and HFCS—*which attacks the cartilage in the joints.* Then later, over the years, the familiar pain and swelling of the joints develop.

Then too, and as is discussed in more detail later; an excess of fructose in the diet leads to the formation of uric acid. This in turn leads to the creation of sodium urate crystals which form in the joints.

The Evidence Is All Around You
—Chapter 9

**Some people dream of being healthy;
others wake up and make it happen.**

Anon

To understand, and hence come to believe that what has been said about sugar is factual—in that it is the number one cause of arthritis—all you need do is observe the evidence all around you. Do this silently and without any fanfare: simply by observing the eating habits of your family members, friends and close acquaintances.

Monitor, in particular those you know who are diabetic, overweight, and generally unhealthy—or who suffer from arthritis. If you do not have the opportunity to watch how they eat, you could find an opportunity to enquire in a 'round about and impersonal sort of way' if they enjoy chocolate, or eat sweets, etc.

In addition, you can listen for supporting evidence which is presented on the TV or in the media generally. Some 12 odd years ago, on TV news, there was a report of a new tribe of people having been discovered in the jungles of a country in the Far East. Up to that time, these natives had remained totally untouched by our civilization.

The presenter went on to say that the doctors and scientists examining these people had been amazed to find they were all totally cancer free. Concluding the news item, he reported that the scientists had stated the situation would probably change once this tribe adopted a Western diet.

Over the years, as we have encountered people with ailments and who were put in our path so to speak: salient points were noted as personal reminders to abstain from refined carbohydrates. These case studies are presented below both as supporting evidence and to show how easy it is to collect such data. However, please note the initials used bear no relation to any person:

A.E. was a lady who would attend Church services on a daily basis. Your heart would reach out to her as she hobbled into Church using two walking sticks. It seemed very likely she was seriously afflicted with arthritis.

After reading Alexander's book—and having personally experienced the cures—we just had to 'risk' offering the book to her to read: hoping we would not offend. Fortunately, she seemed grateful when we gave her the book, explaining its purpose: and said she would read it.

A few weeks later she returned the book and confirmed she did have arthritis in both knees, which was the cause of her disability. Then she told us her story! When she was six years old her parents had started a sweet or candy making factory on the farm. As children they were allowed to eat as much as they wanted and whenever they wanted!

Obviously, reading the book had highlighted the cause of her ailment—we only hoped she would have the resolve to give up the refined carbohydrates, and especially the sweets she had eaten all her life.

G.L. was a consulting engineer, in his early thirties when he first told of his encounter with sugar. At the time he said his wife would buy candy and chocolates and then leave them lying around the office. He found them mouth-watering and could not "keep his hands off them." As the years rolled on he developed arthritis, and would tell us of the different medications he was on. When in his early sixties he had to have both knees replaced.

J.B. was well known to our family. Sometime after reading Alexander's book we heard she had developed arthritis, and was in pain. Because she was miles away on a different continent we could not easily get the book to her. The next best thing was to write a very long email giving a summary of the causes in addition to the recommendations to recover one's health.

She replied saying she was touched by all the love that had prompted the writing of such a lengthy letter explaining the dangers of sugar: but that she *had a long love affair with chocolate* going back many years. Her email said she could never give it up!

Eight years later she had a hip replacement because she could not sleep at night due to the pain, the arthritis was causing. To this day she is on medications to help her with the pain and inflammation.

M.K. was on retirement at the time of our first meeting. His wife worked in a relative's business and we got to meet him through her. He was frequently ill, often needing medical attention. At one stage he needed a ride to hospital for a consultation he had made with a doctor; so we volunteered to take him.

On the return trip we stopped at a restaurant for a cup of coffee. What I remember most from that coffee break was trying not to let the expression of horror show on my face as he *ladled the sugar* into his coffee. Truthfully, I did not know one could or would want to put seven teaspoons of sugar into a coffee.

Over the next few brief years one could not help but notice, that in addition to the sugar in coffee, he went for all the sweet desserts and puddings after meals. To make a long sad story brief—over the short span of the years we knew him he had both knees replaced and then one hip. He was on a waiting list to have the other hip replaced when he died from cancer.

K.N. is a person who loves chocolate-chip cookies, and deserts and sweets in general. He has had a knee replacement and is considering having the other done because of the pain.

T.Q. and B.H are both ladies who cannot walk up the stairs easily because of the pain in their legs and hips. It is not only the 'sweet stuff' that they love to eat—but the other things they do that bring on arthritis. (These causes are mentioned in Chapters 12 and 16 below.)

S. P. was a lecturer on a log-home building course. During his lectures he frequently mentioned his weakness for a popular brand name of doughnuts and said if ever one wanted to make him happy then to give him a gift of them. (The types of dough-nuts he liked are covered with sugar icing or frosting.)

Towards the end of the course he shared with the class his affliction of arthritis; and the pain in his knees which had become so intense it seemed likely he might have to have knee replacements.

N.T. is a fellow who meets regularly with a group of friends. He always has candy on his person—and has a passion for ice-cream. He suffers very much from arthritis in the knees.

K.T. is in her late forties and 'absolutely loves' candy and chocolate. She will forfeit healthy food; so as not to put on weight, but allow *space* for the eating of candy. From what she says the familiar sounding pain is beginning in her knees, and so are varicose veins in her legs.

The above case studies are provided to show the evidence is truly all around—and that it will not be difficult for you to ver-ify the fact that sugar and refined carbohydrates are exceedingly harmful. So *keep an eye out* to confirm you are on the right track and to bolster your determination to proceed with staying healthy.

Happily, not all is sadness. In 2012, we met with a lady real-tor in Florida. She was in her early 70's, as she later divulged; but in extremely good health and very slim. We met with her early one morning, and she worked tirelessly—so much so that by lunch time she looked as if she had not yet started work. Later in the day we commented on this in a complimentary sort of way: saying we just had to ask her secret.

Her reply was rather unexpected, and went something like, "I am 72 years old. I play cards regularly with a group of friends to keep my brain sharp. However, there is no sugar in my house—or anything that contains sugar! Of course if I go to a wedding reception or something like that I will have a piece of wedding cake to be sociable. But other than that I strictly avoid the stuff."

L.B. is an elderly gentleman of 89 years, who joins a group of friends to play cards. He is amazingly fit for his age and we were told how he had assisted his nephew build a concrete wall in his garden. Recently, we had the opportunity to ask his *secret.* And he replied briefly saying, "Eat plenty vegetables and some fruit; along with fish, chicken and meat. *No sugar and no sodas!*"

Beyond Absolute Common Sense —Chapter 10

Tell me and I'll forget. Show me,
and I may not remember.
Involve me, and I'll understand.
Native American Proverb

Because one is surrounded by people who consume sugar containing foods, and drink sodas containing HFCS—the *sharper* your common sense—the greater will be your will-power in resisting what is bad for you.

One does exercises to keep the body healthy and toned. With the same thought, here is an exercise you can do—except this is to increase wisdom and common sense!

The next time you serve up your dinner, comprising healthy and deliciously prepared steak or fish, along with portions of natural and nutrient containing vegetables: set the meal down on a table. Alongside place an empty plate. And pour onto it a generous amount of plain white sugar crystals—say, a similar amount as the food you have on your dinner plate.

As you view both plates compare the healthy life giving food with all its body repairing and maintaining nutrients: against those white crystals that are pure *negative calories*. In looking at the healthy food think to yourself how nourishing it is: then while observing the sugar crystals let it *be indelibly imprinted on your mind that they bring bad health to your body.*

From all the research to date, in my opinion (IMO), the sugar is more than just empty or negative calories—it is an extremely harmful substance. And it is only because of the body's inbuilt healing and survival mechanism—along with the fact other nutrient bearing foods are also eaten—that it can take many years before the harm done becomes evident. Moreover, because the ailments happen so slowly, and in some instances only after people have been consuming sugar for so many years—they are not aware of the link between their ailments and sugar.

For the arthritic especially, but for folk in general, there is 'grim news' in that sugar is the proverbial wolf in sheep's clothing! Because it tastes so 'sweet,' *what is totally hidden from the consumer is the fact that sugar has an exceptionally strong "acid forming effect" within the body.*

As stated in Chapter 8, Dr. Johnson (ref.8) has shown conclusively that the fructose part of sugar causes an increase in uric acid in the blood. Researching the effects of uric acid we looked at the website of the Gout and Uric Acid Education Society (ref.43). They state clearly that when the uric acid levels reach an abnormally high level then sodium urate crystals form in the joints.

IMO that is like pouring sand into your joints: while expecting them not to wear out.

Now you have the answer!

The cause of the deterioration of the cartilage in the joints—is an excessive intake of acidic forming foods and substances—in particular HFCS and sugar.

Therefore the arthritic needs to restrict her intake of overly acidic forming foods—*especially avoiding sugar and HFCS.*

If you read on a 12oz can of coke, this is what is printed under contents:

"Carbonated Water, High Fructose Corn Syrup, Caramel Color, Phosphoric Acid, Natural Flavors, Caffeine, Sugars 39g"

As mentioned earlier 39gm of HFCS equals 1.4ozs or roughly 6½ teaspoons. If you want to be scientific spoon out onto a side plate, or saucer, 6½ teaspoons sugar—it is something to behold just how much sugar that is!

Also note that cola is made from phosphoric acid.

When I was young I mistakenly thought it must be good for me. Imagine the 'let-down' when you discover it is actually bad for you? *That it has an adverse effect on your body's calcium, thus affecting your bones and teeth?* To get to the point William Dufty (ref.20 p.178) quotes Dr. Clive McCay and says the acidity of cola beverages is *about the same as vinegar.* Obviously, it is the amount of sugar in the can which masks this fact, or you would be aware of the acid taste.

William Dufty (ref.20 p.178) and Alexander (ref.2 p.83) both refer to Dr. McCay's original pronouncement concerning his experiment of putting human teeth into a cola beverage—and found they started to soften and dissolve [in the phosphoric acid] within a short time. The original assertion from Dr. McCay regarding teeth dissolving in cola is on many websites.

Then too, it keeps getting worse.

The sugar causes the intestinal wall to deteriorate. While he is not alone in making this statement, Alexander (ref.2 p.89) claims that an over-abundance of sugar throughout your life causes the walls of your intestines to degenerate.

The thing about it is when the intestinal wall deteriorates, it starts malfunctioning. This means it cannot properly absorb the vitamins and nutrients—even if they are in the food being digested. So on the one hand the body has to "find" what nutrients and vitamins it can, to process the sugar through chemical reactions: but on the other—because of the ill effect the sugar begins to have on the intestinal wall—it cannot fully absorb the nutrients and vitamins it so desperately needs.

To add insult to injury, while the sugar is *busy weakening* the intestinal walls; it simultaneously harms what goes on inside the intestines. Dr. Mercola (ref.17) has reported on the fact that sugar persistently destroys the good or friendly gut bacteria; so essential to help with the complete digesting of the food and for the production of some essential vitamins inside the intestines.

There is growing supporting proof for what he claims in many quarters. Recently there was an excellent article on *Gut Bacteria* that appeared in the "Mail on line—UK" Friday 6/14/13 (ref.24). The journalist in turn had condensed it from the book "Cooked" by Michael Pollan, and published by Allen Lane, UK:

From their article, we learn that Michael Pollan narrates, how in the early 2000s, researchers discovered hundreds of new species of bacteria in the human gut doing all sorts of unexpected and helpful things. Saying perhaps their most important function is to maintain the health of the gut wall, or epithelium.

They confirmed that 'gut bugs' manufacture essential vitamins (including vitamin K as well as several B vitamins) and a great many other compounds scientists are only just beginning to recognize.

In the article (from the book) they state that in the Western diet, with its refined carbohydrates, highly processed foods, and lack of fresh vegetables—foods are preserved by killing bacteria [it is like they are sterilized], thus we deprive our gut bacteria of much that is good for them.

If you are serious about maintaining your health, you will not willfully want to *kill off* your friendly gut bacteria. Rather, the arthritic will want to nurture them by eating yogurt (plain and without sugar) and fermented foods; or by taking supplements.

As recently as Thursday, April 25, 2013 we read in *The Irish Times* (ref.25), how the work of Dr Dora Romaguera, from Imperial College London, and his team had highlighted the fact that sugary drinks raise diabetes risk. We then did a Google search and found the doctor's report on various websites.

It seems every extra can of soda pop or cola, consumed in a day, increases the chances of having diabetes by 22 percent when compared with drinking one can a month or less. The scientists reported in the journal Diabetologia that "This study corroborates the association between increased incidence of type-2 diabetes and high consumption of sugar-sweetened soft drinks in European adults."

The crux of Dr Dora Romaguera's report was that, *"Given the increase in sweet beverage consumption in Europe, clear messages on its harmful effect on health should be given to the population."*

Another official who has recently given a clear warning: this time to the people of Holland is Paul van der Velpen, who is head of Amsterdam's health service. If you Google, Paul van der Velpen—*Sugar is most dangerous drug of our time and should come with health warnings;* you will see the news given on several websites (ref.15).

However, to give Emma Innes of the Daily Mail (ref.15) full credit; we first saw a mention of Dr. van der Velpen's comments in her excellent article. It seems that Dr. van der Velpen is concerned with the obesity statistics in Holland where one in two adults are overweight; and as many as one in seven children. Notwithstanding he is also alarmed at the health risks and is quoted as saying, *"Just as with smoking labels, soft drinks and sweet products should come with the warning that sugar is addictive and bad for the health."*

Other Supporting Proof
—Chapter 11

When you discover how little you know,
is the beginning of Wisdom.
                                        Don Slater

1. The Island Where People Forget to Die

We were attracted to the headlines *"The Island Where People Forget to Die"* from a New York Times Magazine article, and wondered if it would have something to say about longevity and retaining health.

It did, in fact telling the story of a Greek man who had recovered totally from serious life threatening cancer—he had been given only nine months to live when in his early 60's—and had then lived to 100. The editor had written his article based on the work of author Dan Buettner, and his own account of the story is in his book *The Blue Zones* and published by the National Geographic Society (ref.7).

We were so intrigued we ordered a copy of the book from Amazon.com and found the story in Chapter 6. This chapter tells the story of a Greek war veteran, named Stamatis Moraitis, who came to the United States in the 1940's. He had come from Ikaria, a small island in the Aegean Sea, off Greece. We estimate he was in his early thirties at the time, got married to a Greek woman and had three children.

Then in his 60's he was diagnosed with terminal cancer, which was confirmed by various other doctors. Rather than undergo chemotherapy in the US, he opted instead to return to his place of birth, the island of Ikaria off Greece, to die there in peace. A decisive factor in his decision making was that the cost of the funeral there would be $200 versus the $1,200 in the US —meaning there would be more money left for his wife.

Arriving at Ikaria he switched to a Mediterranean diet devoid of the highly processed foods available in the US. And he drank red wine each day.

Surprisingly, he did not die as expected. Instead he grew healthier and stronger—eventually living to 100. From our investigation point of view, we needed to know, "As part of his new diet—*did he give up the sugar?*"

Consequently, we so sifted the story to establish whether his sugar consumption had dropped! Then we discovered it had, although not completely—by moving to Ikaria he now only consumed about 25% of what he had formerly done. Largely, as best we could ascertain, because it was not readily available and not really part of the Ikarian diet. Something else of interest was the information that Ikarians eat six times as many beans than people in the US, and it seems they eat them on a daily basis; as well as potatoes.

Amazingly, Moraitis never went through chemotherapy, took drugs or sought therapy of any sort. All he did was move home to Ikaria—and there outlived the doctors who had diagnosed his cancer.

There are nine stories or lessons for 'living longer' in the second edition of Dan Buettner's book *The Blue Zones* that is published by the National Geographic Society (ref.7). You will find them enlightening and interesting.

2. The Mediterranean Diet

Wanting to read more on the Mediterranean diet we did a Google search and came across a Reuter's article written by reporter Genevra Pittman, February 26, 2013 (ref.29). What was so informative was the comparison between different types of diets on 7,500 people, in a study in Spain.

A third of the people participating in the trials were placed on a low fat diet, while the others were given a diet high in olive oil, nuts, fish and fresh fruits and vegetables.

Dr Miguel Angel Martinez-Gonzalez, who worked on the study, has reported that the people on both Mediterranean diets were 28 to 30 percent less likely to develop cardiovascular disease than those on the general low-fat diet. Dr Martinez-Gonzalez said these findings were good news because overall they showed the way to prevent cardiovascular disease is by means of a good diet.

Dr. Dariush Mozaffarian, who studies nutrition and cardiovascular disease at the Harvard School of Public Health in Boston, commented on the research findings as published in the New England Journal of Medicine (nejm.org February 25, 2013). He said things that are discouraged *are refined breads, sweets or candy, and sodas.* He maintained it is a combination of more of the good things and less of the bad things that is so important.

We recommend you access the full article. To access it type in *Dr Martinez-Gonzalez Mediterranean diet* in the Google search engine (ref.29). His findings were posted at an opportune time for us as IMO they illustrate the advantages of discarding the low fat diet idea; in addition to sugar and the refined carbohydrates.

3. The Gerson Miracle
Dr. Max Gerson and his cure for cancer and other diseases

You can obtain the book "The Gerson Miracle" from the Gerson Institute (ref. 28). Though, an easier way to get the overall theory behind the cures he achieved during his lifetime is to rent the movie *The Gerson Miracle* from Netflix. The following are some notes made while viewing the movie:

1. Cancer rates are *one in two* in industrialized nations— or some other chronic disease awaits us—*such as arthritis.*
2. July 1, 1946: Dr. Gerson testified before the US Senate along with five of his cured cancer patients. It was the first time in history a cure had been found for cancer.

3. 1958: The book *A Cancer Therapy by Dr. Max Gerson* detailing studies of cured patients was released. When he died in 1959 he was tracking over 1,500 cured patients.

4. 1977: The Gerson Institute was opened in San Diego by his daughter Charlotte.

5. About 1980/3 Charlotte opened the Tierano Mexico Hospital to treat patients. Laws in the US prohibit treatment for cancer except through radiation, chemotherapy or surgery. [In 2012 a law was passed stating that the drug companies could not be sued for the ill effects arising from Chemotherapy.]

6. The Gerson therapy has highlighted that a change in diet cures asthma. Their suggested diet comprises organic vegetables, fruits and salads (apples seemed to feature largely in the diet).

7. *Sugar is totally eliminated from the diet.*

8. Biological (supplements) that are prescribed, depending on the patient's condition are—Potassium Gluconate, Potassium Acetate and Mono-potassium Phosphate in equal amounts (Product of The Key Company St. Louis), plus Niacin 50 (Nicotinic Acid).

9. Sodium attacks and destroys Potassium.

10. Flax oil is described as the miracle oil. It is recommended as an essential part of the fats in diet. [A word of caution here is not to take flax oil without increasing your intake of vitamin E, as is mentioned in Chapter 22.]

11. The therapy restores proper function of the brain—giving patients a positive rather than a negative outlook to

outside stimulus or events. They experience life to the fullest and do not attempt to heal the body without the soul. (This is also advocated by Hippocrates.)

12. *The body is miraculously designed—it is a forgiving machine that can overcome decades of abuse.* Efficient rest is essential so the body can replenish itself and cure any disease or maintain your health.

The above notes are provided to give an overview—*along with the supporting proof for what the body can achieve once it is spared from having to process the harmful sugars and refined foods.*

There is so much more in the movie. And we recommend it. Especially interesting are the interviews with patients who were cured.

4. Killing Cancer

The latest research on the hazards of sugar was published as recently as Friday June 21, 2013. Lori Johnson is a CBN News Reporter (ref.31) and it was she who penned the original exciting article. In it she tells the story of Dr. Fred Hatfield who had been given three months to live by his doctors, because of his cancer. He had the diagnosis confirmed by three different doctors.

She goes on to say that while Dr. Hatfield was preparing to die, he heard about an anti-cancer diet. Not happy with the idea of using the established cancer treatment route; he decided to give the diet a try—and was very pleasantly surprised to find it worked. *The cancer was cured!*

And that was over a year ago at the time of Ms. Lori's article.

What we gathered from the article is that the diet Dr. Hatfield went on is known as the ketogenic diet and you can obtain more information by visiting the Charlie Foundation at their website (ref.32). From our standpoint we were interested in their stance on sugar—*and sure enough it was taboo!* It seemed the diet recommends the cutting out of carbohydrates so as to 'starve' the cancer cells.

They also classify natural oils such as in olive oil, avocados, and nuts as wholesome food. While on the other hand they strongly warn you should stay away from margarine and any oil that is hydrogenated.

Ms. Lori Johnson's full article is very enlightening and you can access it at CBN's website (ref.31).

5. A Chemo-free Survivor's Health Blog

We providentially stumbled upon an article by Anthony Gucciardi (ref.26), telling the story of a young man, Chris Wark, who was diagnosed with cancer. What was unique about the information was that after his diagnosis—he opted not to go for the conventional chemotherapy treatment. In fact he declined all treatment: concentrating instead on his diet.

The article was so educational we purposely visited Chris' own website (ref.30). It appears that when Chris was diagnosed he had *stage 3 colon cancer.* And he was given a 60 percent chance he could be kept alive for a further five years on chemotherapy.

Because the cancer had spread far beyond the colon itself—including his lymph nodes—Chris, at 26 years of age faced a nightmare decision: and decided to forgo the treatment, concentrating instead on his diet. He did this after his own research into cancer formation—and came to the conclusion nutrition is virtually at the heart of all disease.

Now, nine years later Chris is alive and well and keeps his website up to date, writing frequently on progress and reporting to those who follow his story. In his own words from his website he has this to say:

"The human body is intelligently designed to heal itself, and given the proper nutrients and care, it will. Despite what doctors may have told you, you have options. You have the power to transform your health. If I did it, you can too!"

Reading the article, we gathered Chris had gone to juicing his raw vegetables; but there was no mention regarding sugar, or whether he had given it up. Luckily Chris had a contact email address on his blog (ref.30). So I emailed him, asking if he had excluded the sugar from his new diet.

Chris was so kind as to reply: *he assured me the sugar had been totally excluded when he started his new diet!*

You should access his website and read his truly amazing story and his progress to date. I am sure he maintains it so as to encourage others.

These factual accounts, in this Chapter, of people being healed through eliminating sugar and refined carbohydrates from their diets have been included as sources of *supporting proof* or encouragement for you. If their illnesses could be cured by proper and wholesome food, how will you doing likewise help your arthritis and general wellbeing?

Another Cause Of Arthritis —Chapter 12

Old age is like a bank account.
What you withdraw in later life depends
on what you deposited along the way.

Anon

The lower abdomen probably contains the most important organs in the body because it is these that must process, and obtain all the bodily nutrients and vitamins necessary to care for all the other organs. Yet strangely, they seem to receive the least attention and care.

In his book Alexander (ref.2) is rather forceful in suggesting that one puts an enormous load on the digestive system when drinking at mealtimes. His argument makes sense. By filling your stomach with liquids you dilute the enzymes and gastric juices and acids which are working at digesting the food in the stomach. And not only does the intake of liquids weaken the acids—water and oils are not compatible. Water also breaks down oils making it hard for them to be processed and absorbed; bearing in mind the joints need these oils.

A most amazing syndrome is when one enters a restaurant in USA. Almost the moment you are seated a large glass of iced water is placed in front you! It is the generally accepted custom to drink copious amounts of liquids with one's meals.

Overall, if one drinks liquids on an empty stomach—10 minutes is the minimum time the stomach needs *to empty* or absorb the liquids. You are safer at 15 or more minutes—but try to drink your coffee or wine at least 10 minutes before eating.

If you must drink at mealtimes (old habits die hard) Alexander recommends whole milk: mainly because he sees whole milk as a complete food that will help the arthritic.

Regarding drinking after meals he suggests waiting three hours after an ordinary meal, and up to four hours if a great deal of meat has been eaten. This may initially seem an excessively long time. Therefore, in the beginning even if you can wait two hours before drinking liquids is better than none. Always be conscious of *assisting the digestive process* within you. And when you drink—*drink slowly*: to help your stomach adjust.

Sally Fallon in *Nourishing Nutrition* (ref.11 p.53) has this to say on the subject of drinking at meal times:

"Researchers from both East and West warn that excess liquids taken at meals dilute stomach acid and put undue strain on the digestive process. A good rule is to avoid drinking too much liquid from one half hour before a meal to two hours after."

W.R. was a man we met many years ago. Visiting him one evening he was sitting on his porch enjoying a beer. Eventually he told me that his family knew it was a regular routine that he would have three beers every evening. His first would be with his dinner, and the other two thereafter during the evening. He had done so since adulthood and intended to continue his habit.

The last we heard W.R. was in his old age, and in diapers. The bottom line is drinking with meals places an undue load on the pancreas and the body fails to get the best from the food eaten. As a consequence the stomach and intestines gradually lose the ability to work as designed.

The man above, like most people, had never been told of the harm he was doing over the long term. However, for me, abusing my body by drinking coffee with meals; there was simply no excuse. I knew from previous experience, and had witnessed the results after following the advice from Alexander. But I had so focused on the sugar and the other harmful stuff that I had not given sufficient importance to the necessity of not drinking with meals. It is so easy when one is well once again to become blasé and be tempted to be like everyone else—and I began drinking several cups of coffee at mealtimes. When arriving in the USA it was easy to fall into the coffee habit at breakfast: especially as it tasted so good to drink about three cups per sitting. Drinking coffee at other mealtimes also became a habit.

Consequently the arthritis returned after about six years of such abuse. Therefore, I can personally vouch that drinking liquids with your meals induces arthritis over a period of time.

Suffice to say, now that the message is clear—I refrain from drinking at mealtimes.

To acquire a brief idea of how the stomach works, visualize the shape of a small sausage balloon. Now instead of the rubber in the balloon imagine the walls comprise different layers of muscle. It also has muscles at the opening to the stomach and at the exit to the small intestine.

When you swallow, the muscles at the entry relax and allow the food or drink to enter: then they close. That is when the stomach begins its work. The muscles contract and relax in different motions moving the contents around rather vigorously. The stomach muscles require energy to do all this work that often lasts three to four hours after each meal.

In addition to the muscular actions of the stomach, and to aid in the digestion of the food, gastric juices are 'pumped' into the stomach. These juices contain hydrochloric acid to help in breaking down protein such as meat, fish, etc.; along with other digestive enzymes to help break down other foods.

The stomach, to the best of its ability, turns the contents into a thin liquid. When ready, it releases this liquid, in stages, into the small intestine by relaxing the muscle at the bottom of the stomach at the entry to the intestines. In the intestines the nutrients and goodness is extracted and absorbed into the bloodstream and these are taken to the liver for processing.

The body needs water. It is essential and the question often asked is how much? The general rule is to drink about eight glasses of fluids a day. But this is wide-ranging as it depends on the person's size and weight in addition to ambient temperature and the type of work being done. Fortunately, the body is designed to let you know when it requires water; as when you become thirsty.

A shortage of water leads to constipation and things like a dehydrated skin. On the other hand a really excessive intake of water can be harmful as it places an undue load on the kidneys. So learn to *listen* to your body.

In attempting to observe the rule of not drinking with meals one must *anticipate and plan* when to drink fluids. A guide is to have a beverage on awakening and then a glass of water soon after—but at least 10 minutes before breakfast. You will need to drink again before lunch and dinner and then sometime in the evening.

Chickens And Arthritis
—Chapter 13

Seek wisdom, not knowledge.
Knowledge is of the past,
Wisdom is of the future.
Native American Proverb

If you Google arthritis in animals you will see an array of statistics and facts. It seems that as many as *one in five adult dogs have arthritis—and that even chickens have arthritis.*

Now, in the preceding Chapter we see advanced the argument that drinking water with meals is a cause or arthritis, mainly because it makes digestion difficult and wears out the pancreas thereby resulting in a decrease in the digestive systems ability to extract nutrients. Water is also a great solvent and attacks oils. Just witness how the ocean eventually disperses on its own some catastrophic oil spills that have occurred.

Starting with the chickens! They are reared in coops and their food—chicken pellets, mash, or corn—is placed in trays.

And have you noticed how the drinking water is readily available and placed in a container *alongside the food?*

The chicken takes advantage of the situation—it does not know any better—and immediately after eating it drinks water. Because it is fed mash or pellets it is probably unnaturally thirsty, and drinks more than it would if it was free ranging. It is this constantly drinking water with its food that causes the chicken to get arthritis.

This occurs because chickens were not designed to be fed and watered simultaneously.

The same applies to people and their dogs. When they feed their animals they place the bowl of drinking water alongside the food. So the dogs drink water with their meals.

If ever you have the opportunity look at the National Geographic TV Channel—NatGeoWild—particularly when they are screening programs about animals in Africa: you will notice that none of the animals are struggling with arthritis.

The elephant, giraffe and antelope all walk freely and without pain in their joints. Next observe their water drinking habits. An elephant can drink between 45 to 50 gallons when at the water hole or river—but it does so only once per day *and not while foraging for food.* Sometimes it drinks only every two days. The elephants in the Namibian desert may drink once only every three or four days. Normally, their supply of food is some distance from the water. So elephants *eat without drinking*—after eating they must travel some distance to the watering hole.

Giraffe and antelope as a rule do the same. The water hole is a dangerous place as that is where predators wait in ambush.

Consequently, the antelope only make a daily trip to get water. For them too, their food is some distance from the water: so they eat without drinking water.

The same applies to the guinea fowl (wild birds similar in size to chickens) and to smaller birds. They forage for their food away from the vicinity of water and must drink later; and must make a special trip to do so.

Our domestic farm birds and our pet dogs are robbed of this health benefit, *because they are given water with their meals.*

Undertaking a Google search regarding arthritis in chickens we came upon a woman who we will call K.B. She had at one time set up a website in the hope that some person might help her regarding the arthritis in her chickens.

We were unable to contact K.B. as there was no email or other address on the web page, and the site had been allowed to lapse. But according to K.B. her chickens had arthritis so badly that they would spend the day resting on their hocks; and this onset of the disease occurred after only six months of *"coop living."*

There are other sites about people and their sick chickens. Many seem to think the birds have arthritis because of some viral bacteria and are asking for help and advice. It appears that arthritis in chickens is also a real problem for chicken farmers.

Accordingly, we made contact with a few chicken farmers; in an effort to be of assistance —but mainly to see if they would experiment feeding the birds without water: and then allowing them to drink later. It would have been relatively inexpensive to design and build controlled water drinking points for the birds. And they, and we, would have learnt so much!

Unfortunately, when they heard a book was being written, and no matter the assurance given—they definitely did not want to participate. We could only assume they were afraid there might be some negative publicity. Maybe there was the thought the consumer would cease buying their chickens if made aware they may have had arthritis.

In the meantime it certainly pays to avail of what nature is teaching you: that it is bad for health to drink at meal times. And for those readers with dogs or chickens, you may have found a way to help them as well.

The Essential Oils
—Chapter 14

There's no need to fear the wind
if your haystacks are tied down.
Irish Proverb

Although he does not say so, one can form the opinion that Alexander (ref.2), through his work and research, had unwittingly stumbled upon the fact that the American diet is largely deficient in unsaturated omega-3 linolenic acid oils. We say this because the foods he suggests contain the *right oils* (his terminology: ref.2 p.129), and these are cod liver oil, milk [whole], eggs, butter, fish [mackerel, halibut, salmon, and sardines], and cheddar cheese [not processed]. These foods all contain omega-3 oils, in varying degrees.

He also suggests one should not take things like olive oil and almonds (ref. p.128). It is true that almonds contain omega-6 and eating too many will cause an imbalance in the omega-3 and omega-6 in a diet. However, the latest information also highlights the nutrients available in things like almond nuts are tremendously important, if eaten in moderation.

Then too taking olive oil, as illustrated below, can have special health benefits.

The way to increase omega-3 intake is to eat those foods containing such oils, e.g. meat, fish, eggs: and to take cod liver oil and flax oil, which are rich in omega-3.

In Alexander's book (ref.2 p.163) he suggests taking one tablespoon, equivalent to four teaspoons of cod liver oil each night. However, one has to remember that recommendation was made in the 1970's when the vitamin A and D content of the oils was not so concentrated as today.

At this point in time, there is also a variation in the concentration of the vitamins in different oils. For example, the cod liver oil from Walgreens lists *one* teaspoon (5ml) as containing 4,000 units vitamin A and 400 units vitamin D. The cod liver oil from Seven Seas, U.K., lists under contents that *two* teaspoons (10ml) give 4,000 units vitamin A, 400 units vitamin D, plus 10 units' vitamin E.

It appears, therefore, you get twice the amount of oil by using the Seven Seas oil as against using the Walgreens oil. Consequently, as the arthritic needs the oils, the preferred choice must be that from Seven Seas.

On a cautionary note, one should be careful not to exceed the daily recommended dosages, as vitamin A is stored in the body and an excess is harmful. Walgreens provides this warning on their product:

"Notify a physician if signs of hypervitaminosis A (anorexia, drying or cracking of the skin or lips, irritability, headache, loss of hair) occurs or if signs of hypervitaminosis D (anorexia, nausea, vomiting, weakness, weight loss, diarrhea, vague headaches, stiffness, drowsiness) occur."

The advantage of cod liver oil is its omega-3 content. Two teaspoons of Seven Seas cod liver oil comprises 831mg of eicosapentaenoic acid (EPA), which is an omega-3 fatty acid – plus 939mg of docosahexaenoic acid (DHA), which is also an omega-3 fatty acid, but with a slightly different structure. Both are unsaturated fatty acids (oils). The oil from a bottle is preferred to taking oil capsules.

Dr. van der Merwe, in her book *Health & Happiness* (ref.5 p.133) recommends that the total of vitamin A count should not exceed 10,000 units per day. But in taking oils and vitamins it is always better to err on the cautious side rather than take too much.

It is a preference thing clearly; but our experience with ordinary fish oil has not been great. We tried it as a way of obtaining the omega-3 oils without the vitamin A; but generally many seem to have preservatives added. Moreover, for us, there was no noticeable benefit. In fact some types made one not feel so good.

Regarding cod liver oil Adelle Davis (ref.4 p.118) has said that fish liver oils provide a natural way to obtain sufficient quantities of vitamin D. She has useful advice (ref.4 p.123) on the amount of vitamin D one should take to help with hot flushes for women; with leg cramps, irritability, nervousness and depression. But then she too, also cautions on the danger of exceeding recommended dosages (ref.4 p.120). Excess dosages can cause weakness, fatigue, weight loss, nausea, vomiting, diarrhea, abdominal cramps, headaches, dizziness and demineralization of bones.

However, because vitamin D is such an important vitamin it is worth giving this quote from Adelle Davis (ref.4 p.121), as well as repeating part of it again in Chapter 22:

"Vitamin D can be absorbed into the blood only in the presence of fat. A great increase in rickets has been reported in both the US and Canada because physicians, untrained in nutrition, recommend that infants be given skim milk."

Returning to the essential oils the Gerson Institute (ref.28) has recommended *unrefined* flax oil as a means of obtaining omega-3. The omega-3 content is high in flax seed oil. Whole Foods has a reliable supply, which must be kept refrigerated.

A word of caution, concerning taking the oils! These unsaturated fats, in both cod liver oil and flax oil, *increase the need for vitamin E.* Therefore, a vitamin E supplement should be taken, along with eating those foods high in this vitamin. This information was obtained from Adelle Davis (ref.4 p.139), who says that although the need for vitamin E varies widely—that even a *small increase* in the intake of oils will necessitate an increase in vitamin E.

A guideline setting out the amount of vitamin E one should take is set out in Chapter 22 *Vitamins and Supplements.*

As already mentioned, one of the essential oils is extra virgin olive oil. Wikipedia.org (ref.10) has much to report—here is a short excerpt:

"There is a large body of clinical data to show that consumption of olive oil can provide heart health benefits such as favorable effects on cholesterol regulation and LDL cholesterol oxidation, and that it exerts anti-inflammatory, antithrombotic, antihypertensive as well as vasodilator effects both in animals and in humans. Additionally, olive oil protects against heart disease as it controls the "bad" levels of LDL cholesterol and raises levels of the "good" cholesterol, HDL.

Another health benefit of olive oil seems to be its [ability] to displace omega-6 fatty acids, while not having any impact on omega-3 fatty acids.... This way, olive oil helps to build a more healthy balance between omega-6 fats and omega-3 fats.

Unlike saturated fats, olive oil lowers total cholesterol and LDL levels in the blood. It is also known to lower blood sugar levels and blood pressure.

Olive oil contains the monounsaturated fatty acid oleic acid, antioxidants such as vitamin E and carotenoids, and oleuropein, a chemical that may help prevent the oxidation of LDL particles."

We contacted an olive oil supply company to confirm whether it is safe to cook with extra virgin olive oil. Their customer service representative confirmed you should not use it for deep frying at high temperatures—as it has a low smoke point. Consequently we prefer to obtain our olive oil either on salads or by the teaspoon now and again. Regarding frying; excellent results are obtained by using pure butter.

Further, one needs to be careful when purchasing olive oil as certain suppliers may mix it with other oils such as grape seed or canola oils—and not notify the consumer on the bottle. To check out the genuineness of your olive oil supplier visit the web site of the North American Olive oil Association, Naooa.org. On the site is listed the names of suppliers whose product is guaranteed 100 per cent olive oil.

Dr. van der Merwe (ref.5 p.118) speaks highly of olive oil stating that extra virgin olive oil *contains linolenic acid.* And Sally Fallon (ref.11 p.47) says it has high enzyme content, and:

"Olive oil comprises 75 percent oleic acid; 13 per cent saturated fat; 10 percent omega-6 and 2 percent omega-3. It is a stable monounsaturated fat. Extra virgin olive oil is rich in antioxidants. It is more fattening than butter."

The Guardian, UK, (ref.34) published an article recently by Joanna Blythman and Rosie Sykes titled, *Why Butter Is Good For You.* It was an excellent article extolling the properties of butter. They stated it is an excellent source of vitamins A, D and K, which are essential for the efficient absorption of calcium and phosphorus, and therefore producing strong bones and teeth.

They also said it is rich in linoleic acids; which have significant anti-tumor and anti-cancer actions. They state that butter from grass-fed cows is better than from those fed grain. Overall butter is a wise choice.

Impressed by the article we did a search and found that Joanna Blythman is also the author of *What (What Not) To Eat,* which is available at Amazon.com.

Concluding, we can say with assurance that butter is an ideal food for the arthritic and the person wishing to maintain health. It is a healthy fat that enables the body to absorb vitamins and one which is good for the joints. Sally Fallon (ref.11 p.20) sums it up adequately:

"Use as much good quality butter as you like, with the happy assurance it is a wholesome—indeed essential—food for you and your whole family."

A Cholesterol Story
—Chapter 15

**Don't throw the baby out
with the bath water**
                        German Proverb

As both Alexander and Dr. Abrahamson extol the benefits of eating eggs at breakfast; both for diabetics and arthritics—the omega 3 oils in the yolk of eggs being of particular importance to lubricate the joints—it is prudent to tell the following story:

In the 1970's it suddenly became the vogue that eating eggs were bad for a person. They were branded as being a cause of high cholesterol, and clogging of the arteries with resultant heart failure. As mentioned in the Introduction I joined a large corporation in 1977, where an interesting and rewarding work relationship developed with Don: whereby together we shared the results of the many hours spent researching how to stay healthy.

Because of our positions within the company we were given a free and complete medical examination, including detailed blood analysis, each year. Consequently we decided to use the data from the blood tests to monitor the effects of what was excluded from, and included in our diet.

Don had meanwhile, come across research from Scandinavia highlighting the fact that eggs were necessary to maintain healthy cholesterol within the body. In fact Adelle Davis mentioned in one of her books, *Let's Eat Right To Keep Fit* (ref.4 p.32)—*that the body produced its own cholesterol and an insufficient intake could upset the cholesterol balance!*

So between us, Don and I decided to continue eating eggs each day—on average I ate two—but that we would monitor our cholesterol readings at the annual medical exam. As a result, I can personally report that for the next six years thereafter; my cholesterol readings were perfect.

Since that time eggs have always been part of the daily diet. Based on our experience, they play an important part in maintaining health.

Listed below are the nutrients of one egg as recorded on the egg box cover from *Eggland's Best* (ref.34):

Nutritional Value of One Egg

One Egg	% Daily Value
Total fat 4.5g	7%
Cholesterol 200mg	67%
Sodium 75mg	3%
Protein 7gm	14%

Vitamins	A	6%
	Thiamine	2%
	B2 (Riboflavin)	20%
	B6	4%
	B12	25%
	Folate	10%
	B5 (Pantothenic acid)	15%
	D	20%
	E	30%
Minerals	Calcium	2%
	Iron	4%
	Zinc	4%
	Iodine	45%
	Phosphorus	10%

Plus one egg contains 130mg Omega-3. They claim this high omega-3 content is due to the diet supplied their laying hens.

From their site (ref.34) *Eggland's Best* states their eggs have 3 times more Vitamin B12 compared to ordinary eggs. Just one EB egg will give you 20 per cent of your daily recommended value of Vitamin B12. Not only is vitamin B12 essential in boosting brain power, but it is also needed for the process of converting carbohydrates, fats, and proteins from food into energy.

Vitamin B12 also helps form healthy blood cells, and may aid in the prevention of heart disease. The vitamin B12 found in EB eggs is all found in the rich, bright yolk.

Generally, it appears the diet fed to chickens affects the amount of omega-3 values in eggs. Today, with the stall feeding of cattle and other farm animals there is an excess of animal fats to be sold into the market. If these are added to chicken feed it can only adversely affect the health of the hens and the value of the eggs. *So make sure you buy free range eggs, or eggs with high omega-3 content. Compare the omega-3 value as listed on the different egg boxes, available to you.*

Researching the internet: on their site IncredibleEgg.org state an egg also contains; "Choline 126mg; Selenium 15mcg; and Magnesium 6mg."

Wikipedia.com (ref.10) states quite clearly that the yolks of eggs contain lecithin.

In addition, from their excellent internet site, the *World of Technology* (ref. 16) has an article titled *5 Reasons to Have Eggs for Breakfast* posted. The following is a concise quote:

"Some very specific things about eggs make it the perfect meal for you. Considering breakfast is the most important of the day. The following nutritional aspects of eggs make it your ideal morning meal.

Energy Booster: Eggs can give you that boost of energy which helps you go through the rest of the day. The egg yolk has a lot of healthy fats that make it a storehouse of energy. For best results, eat boiled egg yolk.

Proteins To Strengthen You: You need not only energy but also the strength to carry on with your work for the rest of the day. Egg white has protein called albumin. Having albumin early in the morning helps your body absorb lots of proteins. If you have been working out, it will help build your muscles.

Eggs Help You Lose Weight: Contrary to popular notions. Having eggs for breakfast does not lead to weight gain. Studies done at the Pennington Biomedical Research Centre, in Louisiana USA have found that a breakfast of eggs helps you lose weight. This is because high protein foods are a natural suppressant of hunger.

Eggs Keep You Full: Eggs are actually very filling. If you have an omelet made of 2 eggs in the morning, you will not feel hungry till lunch. This stops you from snacking on unhealthy things in between meals.

Eggs Improve Brain Power: Apart from strength and energy, you also need a sharp brain to make you successful. The nutrition of eggs helps your brain sharpen itself. Choline is a nutrient present in eggs that stimulates the brain into action. It helps improve memory and better cognitive reasoning."

Referring again to Adelle Davis (ref.4 p.101) she states that consuming foods with cholesterol is essential and necessary to health. *And that eating eggs is safe.* They contain vitamin E which is there to process the healthy oils within the egg. On the same page she has this to say which should make those who are afraid to eat eggs take note:

"Furthermore, when no cholesterol is obtained from the diet, the body produces cholesterol far more rapidly than when the intake is high."

Remaining with Adelle Davis (ref.4 p.32) she also says this about the body producing its own cholesterol:

"Studies have shown that approximately 800 milligrams of cholesterol are obtained daily from a diet high in animal fat. A normal adult liver produces 3,000 milligrams or more per day. Cholesterol forms the raw material from which vitamin D, the sex and adrenal hormones and bile salts are made. The fact that cholesterol is concentrated in such vital tissues as the brain and nerves indicates that it serves valuable unknown functions in maintaining health."

Sally Fallon in *Nourishing Nutrition* (ref.11 p.12) has much to add about the nutritional value of eggs and this about cholesterol:

"Cholesterol is needed for proper function of serotonin receptors in the brain. Serotonin is the body's natural feel-good chemical. Low cholesterol levels have been linked to aggressive and violent behavior, depression and suicidal tendencies.......Dietary cholesterol plays an important role in maintaining the health of the intestinal wall."

Dr. Joseph Mercola (ref.17) has also written extensively about cholesterol and heart disease on his internet site. Here is a small excerpt:

"Cholesterol is a much debated topic in the medical community. Cardiologists' and big pharmaceutical companies will tell you that lowering your cholesterol keeps your heart healthy. This is why cholesterol-lowering statin drugs are the leading drug category in terms of sales. *But {he warns} drastically lowering your cholesterol levels will increase your risk of dying!*

Your body needs cholesterol in the same way that it needs air and water. Cholesterol is found in every cell of your body and is involved in important processes, including the production of bile acids, cell membranes, hormones, and vitamin D."

Another person who writes about cholesterol on her informative internet site is Margaret Durst (ref.18). Here is a short and very important quote:

"Before banning cholesterol, consider its beneficial functions in the body. These include production of hormones for balancing blood sugar levels, for regulating mineral levels, and for promoting healing and balancing the tendency towards inflammation. Cholesterol is vital to proper nerve function. It plays a key role in the formation of memory and the uptake of hormones in the brain, including serotonin, the body's feel-good chemical. Cholesterol is the precursor to vitamin D and bile salts used for the digestion of fats. It is also an important component of cell membranes which help differentiate the inside of cells from the outside of cells. Cholesterol is also the body's repair substance—scar tissue contains high levels of cholesterol."

When people ceased eating eggs they certainly *threw out the baby with the bath water!* By falsely discrediting eggs—people have been denied the very essential vitamins and nutrients, that are in the egg; and which are required by the body to maintain healthy cholesterol balance.

To maintain your health and to combat arthritis one needs this healthy food. The real cause of high cholesterol is the sugar;

the white flour; the polished rice, and the bad fats—notably hydrogenated fats and oils: that people eat in processed food, or in their cooking oils. Adelle Davis (ref.4 p.232) is rather specific about what actually causes increases in cholesterol. One needs to take seriously what she says:

"Hydrogenated fats raise cholesterol."

What Aggravates Arthritis
—Chapter 16

A danger foreseen is half-avoided.
Cheyenne Proverb

<u>Salt versus potassium</u>

Salt is a most necessary and essential element for good health, *and must be part of the diet.* Moreover it serves a useful function in providing flavor to our food. Ask anyone who has ever tried eating meat without salt.

The harm comes from eating too much!

On a TV news broadcast there was a sad story of a grief stricken young couple whose very young baby had died because of too much salt in its diet. It turned out the couple were struggling financially and could not afford baby formula for the child—so had used corn flakes to feed their baby. The salt content in the corn flakes was so high the child died.

Evidently adults can handle excess amounts of salt far better; but not without consequences. It has been reported that patients with high blood pressure, on average, consume too much salt. Many authors have stated that arthritics too, have an affinity for salt.

How does excess salt affect the arthritic?

As best we can ascertain it upsets the balance of other essential minerals.

In this regard it is a good idea to turn directly to Dr. Mercola (ref.17):

"As mentioned earlier, another important factor that needs to be taken into account is the potassium to sodium ratio of your diet. *Imbalance in this ratio* can not only lead to hypertension (high blood pressure) but also contribute to a number of other diseases, including……. heart disease and stroke: memory decline: osteoporosis: ulcers and stomach cancer: kidney stones: cataracts…… *and rheumatoid arthritis!"*

You may wish to research how much salt to consume daily, on Dr. Mercola's site.

To sum up: *excess* salt, or sodium chloride, causes a deficit of potassium in the body. Potassium is an absolutely necessary nutrient. So how then does one restore the correct sodium to potassium balance? It is a bad idea to think of taking potassium supplements! Luckily, the manufacturers of potassium supplements warn about this—and that one should only do so under a medical practitioner's direction.

This is where a 'thank you' is due Dr. Mercola. It was in one of his articles where he wrote that the best way to increase one's potassium is by eating those foods most rich in the mineral, viz.

lima beans, winter squash, broccoli, asparagus, cooked spinach and avocado. By increasing potassium levels with these natural foods it removed the cause of my leg cramps and *restless leg syndrome.*

Formerly, eating bananas seemed the best way to obtain potassium. That was before reading Dr. Johnson's book *The Sugar Fix* (ref.8). Now we are aware it is a bad idea to eat too much fruit as it raises one's fructose levels too high.

Dr. Mercola (ref.17) warns one should avoid processed foods—as these are normally loaded with salt for flavor, but in addition they may also contain fructose. He says:

"To reiterate, processed foods are also loaded with fructose, which is clearly associated with increased heart disease risk, as well as virtually all chronic diseases."

They are loaded with fructose to make them flavorful and edible. Fructose is cheaper than sugar, besides it extends the shelf-life of the product. But it is not good for you!

We once had the opportunity to view horses eating in a livery stable on a sugar cane plantation. As all the fields were cultivated with sugar cane there was virtually no grass for the horses. To provide them with 'greens' the people in charge would organize the cutting of cane tops and place these in the feeding troughs. As a means of encouraging the horses to eat the tops they poured molasses all over them—much like people pour syrup over their pancakes.

The fructose in processed foods hides the fact they actually do not taste so good.

Before leaving potassium, one will benefit tremendously from this important piece of information attributable to Dr. Mercola (ref.17):

"Why is potassium so important? Among other things, your body needs potassium to maintain proper pH levels in your body fluids, and it also plays an integral role in regulating your blood pressure. It's possible that a potassium deficiency may be more responsible for hypertension than excess sodium. Potassium deficiency leads to electrolyte imbalance, and can result in a condition called hypokalemia. Symptoms include: water retention, raised blood pressure, heart irregularities, muscular weakness and muscle cramps."

Final words on salt—do not buy salt which contains chemicals to make it *free running*. Some of these chemicals are really damaging to health over the longer term. Read the ingredients carefully. Buy a good quality sea salt which is chemical and preservative free. Good brands are Lima—Atlantic Sea Salt, and Himalayan Salt.

Milk

Milk is good for you!

An aggravation is the lack of a supply of *nourishing whole milk.*

Alexander (ref.2 p.51) describes nutritious whole milk as a complete food, because of the cream which he describes as one of the right oils to lubricate joints—and is essential to the arthritic. In fact the benefits of milk are all acclaimed by Adelle

Davis (ref.4), Sally Fallon (ref.11), Dr. Mercola (ref.17) and Dr. Abrahamson: as well as by other reputed researchers.

Actually, Dr. Richard J. Johnson (ref.8 p.196) lists a further benefit when speaking about the kidneys. He says a normal function of the kidneys is to take uric acid out of the blood and eliminate it through the urine. However, they will perform this function more efficiently *if one drinks plenty of milk and consumes other dairy products.*

How many older people are still alive who remember how milk was delivered when they were children? It arrived in glass bottles—and after standing in the refrigerator for a while; the cream would separate out and rise to the top where it was clearly visible.

In those days you only had whole milk or skim milk—the latter from which the cream had been removed; for making butter, or for sale as cream.

Then milk producers devised the concept of homogenizing milk. To homogenize milk it is forced at high pressure through tiny orifices. This breaks up the fat globules in the cream to such a small size that they remain suspended in the milk—and no longer rise to the top.

To homogenize milk means an extra operation in the packaging process. This means an increased cost. So you ask, "What is in it for them—remembering the profit motive."

The first benefit is it makes the milk *look extra white* when packaged in plastic bottles. This applies equally to the 1 percent milk and 2 percent milk—in fact, once homogenized, these do not look *watered down.* Therefore, they resemble whole milk when standing on the shelf in the refrigerator in the grocery store.

The marketing strategy was extremely clever when suppliers termed the 1 percent and 2 percent varieties *as low fat milk* instead of, say, *reduced cream milk* which it is. In marketing it is what the consumer "hears" that is important!

What the consumer *"heard"* from the low fat milk slogan: was that if he used those varieties he would *lose fat, or weight.* Especially, as the media at that time was extolling the advantages of a low fat diet.

Because they can sell the 1 percent and 2 percent varieties for the same price as whole milk—it is tantamount to getting "free" cream when they remove it from the milk. But then too, it gets even better for the producers. The excess milk produced in summer, when there is plentiful grass, does not go off when it is dried and can thus be stored. It is later used as 1 percent and 2 percent when needed. The homogenization process facilitates the use of dried milk.

Unfortunately the consumer using recycled dried milk can suffer health defects. In the 70's or 80's an American scientist wrote a paper describing how the milk drying process resulted in contaminants forming in the milk that would lead to a *hardening of the arteries.* We lost that original article unfortunately, and no amount of searching the internet would bring it to light. However, we luckily stumbled on it in Sally Fallon's *Nourishing Nutrition* (ref.11 p.35). She has the necessary supporting literature referenced in her bibliography, and below is a short quote:

"Powdered skim milk is added to the most popular varieties of commercial milk – 1% and 2% milk. Commercial dehydration methods oxidize cholesterol in powered milk, *rendering it harmful to the arteries.* High temperature drying also creates......and nitrate compounds which are carcinogens [toxic substances aiding cancer]... as well as free glutamic acid which is toxic to the nervous system."

The other thing about 1 percent and 2 percent milk is that contrary to popular belief—rather than helping one to lose of weight—according to Alexander (ref.2 p.53), it has the reverse effect and causes the consumer to *put on weight.*

Regarding the pasteurization of milk, there is this quote from Sally Fallon (ref.11 pp.34-35):

"Pasteurization destroys all the enzymes in milk...these enzymes help the body assimilate calcium. That is why those who drink pasteurized milk may suffer from osteoporosis...... Modern pasteurized milk, devoid of its enzyme content, puts an enormous strain on the body's digestive mechanism....... The result is allergies, chronic fatigue and a host of degenerative diseases."

To maintain optimum health one's first choice is to find a source, say your local farmers market, where you can purchase raw milk (milk direct from a reputable farmer, which has not been pasteurized or homogenized). That way you get all the vitamins and minerals as intended by nature. It is something to think about—milk contains what it does, including all the cream, for its proper assimilation and absorption. The cream is necessary for utilizing and 'burning' the carbohydrate, and the vitamins and nutrients are necessary for the chemical reactions as the body utilizes this health giving food.

If raw milk is not available; then attempt to purchase milk which has been pasteurized but not homogenized.

Breakfast cereals

These generally fall under processed foods. Some cereals are so loaded with sugar frosting it is as good as eating candy. Others are so refined and processed they retain little food value. In fact one uses valuable bodily nutrients to process them.

Cereals have become popular because the consumer has been sold on the idea 'of convenience.' In reality there were other various advertizing ploys. One in particular says a certain breakfast cereal will assist in losing weight.

A.K. was a young man who had began putting on weight. He thought it was because a change in his work situation meant he was spending longer hours in a sedentary position in front of his laptop. Consequently, when he saw an advertisement on TV for a particular breakfast cereal that would aid in losing weight; he went along and bought a few boxes.

A week later he became conscious of continual pain in his elbow joints as well as in the joints of his fingers. Reflecting on this new *ailment* and questioning what changes he had made in his diet: he wondered if it might be because he was having the new cereal for breakfast. To evaluate his theory he ceased eating the cereal—and to his surprise the pain in the joints disappeared after one week. He says he was lucky the preservatives, which he assumed had been added to the cereal, acted so quickly he could figure out they might be the cause.

Although it is not stated on the box—cereals must have preservatives added—or some change made to the contents that will deter the bacteria and bugs from causing decay. Where it states 'preservative free' on the box the cereal may well fit into this latter category.

Alternatively, all the goodness may have been extracted from the original grains used to make the cereal. With wheat, for example, if one removes the bran and the wheat germ (the constituents containing the nutrients and vitamins), then what is left will have a prolonged shelf-life as the bugs and bacteria will not consider it edible. This quote from Sally Fallon (ref.11 p.25) gives food for thought:

"Whole grains that have been processed by high heat and pressure to produce puffed wheat, oats and rice, are actually quite toxic and have caused rapid death in test animals."

From research to date, a healthy breakfast cereal is old fashioned oats. The supplier, Quaker Oats, has assured us it is totally preservative free—has not yet been genetically modified —and that in the milling process every effort has been made to retain the bran and the germ.

Chewing

It will not hurt to rewrite an old proverb as—*the way to a man's 'health' {heart} is through his stomach.*

To get the most out of your food you need to chew it properly—it is after all the start of the digestive process—the beginning of extracting all the goodness and nutrients from the food. Especially see it as being 'kind' to your stomach; as taking some of *the load off it.*

When people feel under pressure with too much to do—they can be tempted to *wolf down* a meal. And over time this can become a habit: a way of eating. The net result; the body becomes malnourished as it cannot extract fully all the nutrients in the food eaten. The digestive system just cannot process the food satisfactorily, and much goodness simply passes through.

In addition, with poor chewing, a great load is placed on the stomach walls and the pancreas. One needs to *nurse* those organs and not *wear them out.*

Heredity Ailments
—Chapter 17

The apple does not fall far from the tree
German Proverb

The above German proverb was found on Wikiquote (ref.12). Immediately below it they give an explanation which says that, 'children observe daily [the behavior of their parents]—*and often follow their example.*

Again giving credit where due; it was in Alexander's book (ref.2) where we first saw the argument advanced that children inherit their parent's bad eating habits—thus incurring the same ailments—making it appear as if the health problems are inherited.

It has to be about the most *damming* assertion one can make to suggest that a person has an ailment, or is likely to get it, because your parents and grandparents had it. In this regard we are talking of things like arthritis, diabetes and cancer—not diseases that are transmitted via germs or microbes such as aids.

But to make a false statement about ailments that are self-inflicted; saying they are hereditary—is cruel and dispiriting—because it destroys the hope: that if you alter your habits there is the real possibility you *will not* suffer the same ill health as your parents. Or, that if you do have the same illness—that you can be cured!

A spirit of optimism and hope, if founded on good practice, is necessary and helpful in tackling any infirmity. Helen says it so adequately in this quote:

"Optimism is the faith that leads to achievement.
Nothing can be done without hope and confidence."
Helen Keller

T.T.'s earliest childhood memories of his mother working in the kitchen are of the way she added sugar to their meals. Her favorite vegetable was pumpkin and he can remember her making it super-delicious by adding generous amounts of sugar and butter. Another of his much loved dishes she prepared was a steamed pudding. It consisted of a cake mixture made of white flour and soaked in cane syrup.

Then too his mother always had a supply of candy and chocolate on hand. And he knew from experience that if ever she ran out then he could go visit his grandmother, who lived next door, as she was bound to have a supply. His mother and grandmother shared the same fondness for candy—as indeed so did he by this time.

In a similar way many recipes are passed down from mother to daughter—especially for things like chocolate cakes, cream scones and chocolate chip cookies.

An example of the lack of appreciation of the *cause,* that bad eating habits can be passed on to children, is when you visit to your doctor's office. In completing a general questionnaire you will be asked what ailments your parents and grandparents had—maybe even what they died from. But on such a questionnaire we have yet to be asked, "What did the parents eat and drink?"

In essence it probably stems from a lack of knowledge on the proper use of statistics, and fact gathering, as mentioned in Chapter 1. The way the questionnaires are structured they inadvertently exclude other factors which may in turn have been totally responsible for the sickness.

If you inherit from your parents their incorrect and harmful eating habits (say for example, loads of vanilla ice-cream covered with lots of melted dark chocolate, for dessert each mealtime); and go on to maintain these bad habits and poor lifestyles—then you too are more than likely to end up with the same problems.

Alexander Vindicated —Chapter 18

**The proof of the pudding
is in the eating.**
Irish Proverb

We had heard and read so many positive reviews about Dale Alexander, we were surprised and saddened to read there had been negative comments made about his qualifications —in that a certain honorary doctorate degree may have been awarded after he had made a large donation to a university. And that claims to other qualifications may have been unfounded.

It is important you are made aware of these facts, and for that reason we are thankful to Dr. Gabe Mirkin (ref.37) for reporting them on his website. We came upon his site when doing a Google search titled *cod liver oil and arthritis*. In his paper Dr. Mirkin reports how the Federal Trade Commission [FTC] had investigated Dale Alexander's qualifications and found them not to be correct.

It appears that on September 7, 1956, the FTC also charged that the ads for Alexander's book were *false, misleading, and deceptive.* In addition, from Dr. Mirkin's article, the hearing examiner at FTC decided this about Alexander's book *Arthritis and Common Sense:*

"[It] is but a thesis by Alexander predicated on unsupportable and improvable postulates; and amounts to nothing more than a collection and summation of the author's theories concerning arthritis, rheumatism and related diseases, all of which are pure theory."

Try as we might we could not access the proceedings from that hearing, to obtain a full account. Therefore, we are indebted to Dr. Dr. Mirkin for reporting the FTC actions.

My initial reaction to reading the article was it brought about feelings of great sadness. Indeed it seemed an injustice that the hearing (as far as one can assume) concentrated solely on qualifications—that there was not even the slightest mention, or a review of the great many cases of people being helped with; or who had been cured of their arthritis: or who had left wheelchairs to walk again.

Nonetheless there is encouraging and supporting news in Dr. Mirkin's article as he goes on to tell how Alexander had advocated taking cod liver oil: and that the recent findings, from respected researchers in Berlin, had shown this therapy to be effective. Quoting from the article:

"In this study, 43 patients with rheumatoid arthritis took 1 gram of cod liver oil daily for three months. Fifty-two percent had less morning stiffness, 42 percent had less pain, and 49 percent had less swelling, Sixty-five percent felt that the cod liver oil helped relieve their pain, and 98 percent felt that they could take it in spite of its awful odor."

We suggest you access Dr. Mirkin's website (ref.37) and read his article. The full reference to the Berlin report from which the above quote was obtained is given as (ref.38).

If the German researchers used cod liver oil solely as a treatment or remedy, without any change to diet, then the results are truly amazing. Because, although Alexander advanced the use of cod liver oil as a remedy—he did so with the admonition there be strict adherence to the principle of avoiding those things which brought about the onset of the ailment in the first place.

Wanting to see if there were any other comments, positive or otherwise, we accessed Amazon.com to read the customer reviews for Alexander's book *Arthritis and Common Sense*.

The first is from "Bob in PA" in April 2, 2005:

"This book saved my life! I highly recommend it! 20 yrs ago when I was 30 I could barely walk. I was always in so much pain... every dang joint in my body! Now I am totally healthy at 50!!! The book does talk about exercise... not to do it unless your joints are oiled!! It would be like starting a car without oil... the moving parts would be damaged. Exercise when you're healed! Follow the guidelines in this book & your joints will be oiled! It worked for me! I just wonder where I would be today without my dad giving me this book 20 yrs ago."

The second review is from "A Customer" in August 17, 2000:

"When I was in my mid-20's I was diagnosed with gout. Although I received medication, there wasn't much improvement. Fortunately, my aunt loaned me her copy of this book. Within days, the gout was gone, simply due to following some of the basics in the book. However, what I didn't know was why she believed in this book so strongly. Years before my gout, my aunt had suffered terribly from arthritis. She was so crippled with it that she couldn't even bathe herself. Despite extensive medication, all the doctors could do was help alleviate her pain, but were unable to cure the arthritis, itself. Out of desperation, she bought this book. To everyone's amazement, not only was she able to start taking care of herself again, she started going on walks. Up until the time she died in her 80's, she used to walk for over a mile a day.

The third is from someone using the alias "bmerfeld55" in July 12, 2001. It is a relative of Alexander's:

"When my grandfather wrote this book, my mother was just two years old. I know a lot has changed in the world of medicine and scientific discovery has improved all of our lives, but one constant remains, nothing is better for preventing a problem or solving one than good common sense.

My grandfather was well ahead of his time; his theories teach people that a simple solution is often times the best solution. Now almost 50 years later, evidence and testimonials have proven him to be right, and because it is in all of our best interests to protect our joints and our bodies, take this book home and read through it."

The fourth review is from Angelica B. Yerger in September 16, 2004:

"Whether or not his theories are scientifically correct, the advice in this book produces great results."

The fifth review is from Lady Rybs in July 10, 2010:

"As a young woman in the 1970's my doctor told me he could not help me with my arthritis: that I should go to the library and get a book called, "Arthritis and Common Sense" by Dale Alexander. I purchased a copy. Followed the plan and was up and about in 6 weeks! I have been able to manage my arthritis for 40 years by following this advice.

Now I buy copies and send to my friends that are having a struggle. I always hope and pray that they will get as much benefit from it as I have. I am so glad that it is still available at Amazon.com."

Other folk have posted reviews on Amazon.com which you may wish to research.

Harmful Preservatives
—Chapter 19

If it's drowning you're after,
don't torment yourself
with shallow water.
Irish Proverb

Wikipedia, the free encyclopedia, (ref.10) is a wonderful source of factual and unbiased information. Searching under *preservatives* the site highlights the fact there are two kinds:

Firstly, the natural or *class one preservatives* that can be found in a person's kitchen such as and including vinegar, salt, etc. To which we can add lemon juice and ascorbic acid (a synthetic vitamin). There is no quarrel with class one type preservatives.

Secondly, Wikipedia mentions that "class two preservatives refer to preservatives which are chemically manufactured."

It is the chemically manufactured preservatives which cause the harm! Little do folk realize how much of their suffering can be as a result of repeatedly consuming them in their food or drink. Preservatives may even be found in some medications and vitamin supplements. Consider these personal stories:

L.M. was an elderly man who was taken out for an evening meal by his son and daughter-in-law, to a Chinese restaurant. The following morning he had a blinding migraine.

Subsequent research led him to discover that some Chinese restaurants may add monosodium glutamate (MSG) to *flavor* the food they sell: while other food producers' use it as a preservative.

The network site GraceLinks.org (ref.19) reports that MSG can cause headaches, nausea, weakness, difficulty breathing, drowsiness, rapid heartbeat, and chest pain. The site highlights the fact, and cautions, that MSG may be termed *natural flavor* or *hydrolyzed yeast extract* by some manufacturers. The site goes on to report that nitrites, common preservatives used in cured meats such as sausages, bacon and hot dogs are unhealthy according to a 2006 study.

There is much more to be found on their site regarding harmful preservatives and their research is very good—definitely worth reading.

Matt's story has already been covered in Chapter 3; outlining his years of suffering due to the preservative tartrazine. It is a *no wonder* he is now wary of foods containing preservatives. There are other stories:

D.T. recounts how he and his wife were invited over for an evening meal by a relative. She had prepared a lovely dinner with a chicken type stew as the main course. It was delicious and looked appetizing with a slight 'pink' coloring from the food spices she had added. Complementing the chef, they were informed the spices with the coloring, had *come from a bottle,* already mixed and blended, and had been purchased in the grocery store.

He shared how, on the following morning, he could hardly get out of bed due to the pain in his hips, it was that severe. As he lay there, casting his mind over *what strange or different foods* he had consumed in the previous 24 hours he remembered the chicken flavoring from the night before. The reason for his sudden pain was instantly obvious! He ended by saying, that as he lay there—he wondered how many people ended up having hip replacements if they ate "that stuff" on a regular basis with absolutely no idea or inclination as to the cause of their pain.

V.M. was a woman who told how one of her friends with a small child, who had recently started school, had to take the young fellow to her doctor. It seemed this child suffered as a result of hyperactivity; to such an extent the teachers had requested they seek medical attention for him.

Later, the problem was solved when the doctor identified the cause of the child's hyperactivity as consuming soft drinks containing sodium benzoate, and eating dried fruit preserved with sulphur dioxide. By eliminating these preservatives from his diet the child was on the road to recovery.

A.K. recounted how he was at work in his factory, just prior to a Christmas season, when a young saleslady visited in the hopes of making a sale of items to be used as gifts for loyal customers.

In the ensuing discussion she told A.K. how she had just visited a large sweet manufacturing concern not far from where he was situated. And that these people, having completed their Christmas orders, were now producing for Easter. He told her he was amazed considering that Easter was still some four months away. Her reply was she had made the very same comment to the production manager who had said, "There are enough preservatives in those Easter eggs they will last six years!"

Possibly, a good way to view preservatives, is that they are *poisons* added to food, or beverages, to *"kill off the bacteria"* that would otherwise spoil those items. They vary in intensity as chemicals depending on the type and amount added. The concentrations may be so mild that most people do not discern them as being the cause of their feeling unwell; or may fail to gauge the harmful effects they are having on their health over the longer term.

The body is not designed to *"process chemicals"*—however these are added to food to give the produce a *shelf-life* so as to increase the profitability of the manufacturer.

Preservatives really do affect a person. About 11 years ago B.N. appeared on a TV News broadcast specifically to deliver a personal message. He had suffered all his life with incessant sneezing—and no amount of visits to doctors or the taking of medication had brought him any relief. Now, at his late stage in life, it had been discovered that the cause of the disorder was due to an additive in the breakfast cereal which he had consistently eaten every morning.

As well as not being good for the human body, preservatives have another harmful effect. Because it is so logical to assume that if they *kill off* the bacteria in food and beverages—they are still *doing their work* after they have been consumed: as they make their way through the stomach and intestines. It is there they cause damage that is most harmful—as now they *kill off* the good or friendly bacteria in the intestines!

Dr. Mercola (ref.17), in an excellent article states that people are generally low on *good or friendly bacteria* in their intestines. And that noticeably the shortage is particularly prevalent among people over 60. Therefore, those who may need the nutrition most are losing out as they lack the bacteria to help with the digestion of their food—and the manufacture of essential vitamins. The arthritic needs every bit of nutrient his system can absorb so as to help heal the arthritis and return to health.

The more chemicals, or case two preservatives, that are consumed the greater the damage done to the good or friendly bacteria. In addition they harm the body cells and organs. How else would they cause such things as migraine and other bodily disorders?

Be very, very grateful if you get headaches as a result of eating preservatives. Those headaches are your *health barometer* and will warn you when you have eaten something harmful—they will also remind you to remain vigilant and to shy away from processed foods.

In conclusion, one needs to be wary concerning the listing of some ingredients on food packages. For example the statement on a package which reads *No added Preservatives* means exactly what it says—that no preservatives have been added. However, the ingredients used probably *already contained* the preservatives. A case in point is the oil used to roast peanuts or fry potato chips. The particular oil used will almost certainly contain preservatives, or have been treated in some way, to prevent it from becoming rancid. This oil now also serves to 'preserve' the final product.

A closing word on preservatives is that they cause tremendous *hidden* stress within your body, as it fights the good fight to keep you healthy.

Detrimental To Your Health —Chapter 20

An ounce of prevention is worth a pound of cure!
Irish Proverb

The wording on a bottle of peanut butter in the local grocery store specifically reads:

"This peanut butter is preservative free!
There is no need to refrigerate after opening!"

And one asks, "How can this be?"

How did the manufacturer defeat nature when it is the character of foodstuffs to "go off" and become rancid? When if, for example, you cut an orange into small segments and expose it to the atmosphere—after 10 minutes all the vitamin C will have been oxidized: and the bacteria from the air begins settling on the pieces and starts the process of decay?

You will have noticed how even fruit that is not cut, if left in the fruit basket on the kitchen counter, goes off when not eaten.

So how then does a peanut manufacturer develop that which has continually evaded scientists in their efforts to preserve food? The answer is, in order to improve shelf-life and prevent the product from going off, the manufacturer *works on the oils* in the peanut butter by altering their molecular structure through hydrogenation; i.e. using the gas hydrogen during the processing of the nuts.

The oils are therefore "hydrogenated!"

As mentioned above, the bacteria in the air are governed by instinct. To us the food may look and taste the same—*but the bugs know different!* They will not land on anything which is not food. Therefore they purposely avoid the peanut butter.

Adelle Davis (ref.4 p.33) describes very aptly why the hydrogenated peanut butter does not go rancid:

"When fats are hydrogenated, the hydrogen is added to the unfilled chains of the essential fatty acids; thus their health-building value is destroyed. Such fats can supply calories but nothing more: they cannot become rancid—*neither can they support life of bug or beast.*

Each year the list grows longer—margarine; hydrogenated cooking fats; processed cheeses; and now *peanut butter."*

Just so you know: Whole Foods, in their grains section, have a self-operating machine that will grind peanuts into peanut butter. Making it on their facility ensures there is no hydrogenated oil, or other mineral oils added. Refrigerate on reaching home.

Below are supporting quotes regarding the hazards of hydrogenated oils as given by Sally Fallon (ref.11 p.13 p.15):

"The cause of heart disease is not animal fats and cholesterol but rather a number of factors inherent in modern diets, including excess consumption of vegetable oils and *hydrogenated fats;* excess consumption of refined carbohydrates in the form of sugar and white flour; mineral deficiencies, particularly low levels of protective magnesium and iodine....... Margarine [containing hydrogenated oils] provokes *chronic high levels of cholesterol* and has been linked to both heart disease and cancer."

Because many folk are anxious to lose weight, diet soda pop and colas have gained in popularity. Since there is mounting evidence they are not healthy it was gratifying to come across an article from *The Indianapolis Star* which stated these drinks actually do the opposite to helping lose weight—they add on the weight! The article was titled *Study: Diet Soda Doesn't Help You Lose Weight by* reporter, Shari Rudavsky from The Indianapolis Star; July 11, 2013. (ref.33)

Her story covered the work of Professor Susan Swithers, from Purdue University, who has highlighted the dangers of drinking diet sodas. After reading Shari's article we accessed Purdue University and in the search box typed in *"Study: Diet soda doesn't help you lose weight by Professor Susan Swithers."*

Ms. Swithers found that diet sodas may be linked to a number of health problems from obesity to diabetes to heart disease. One large study found that people who drank artificially sweetened soda were more likely to experience weight gain than those who drank non-diet soda. Others found that those who drank diet soda had twice the risk of developing metabolic syndrome, often a precursor to cardiovascular disease, than those who abstained.

The study included drinks containing aspartame, sucralose and saccharin. About 30 per cent of American adults regularly consume these sweeteners.

When Professor Swithers was asked whether diet sodas are worse for you than regular sodas: her reply was a classic! She said that was the wrong question—that the correct question is, "*What good are sodas for you in the first place?*"

The Professor's report is full of much factual data from her research that is truly worthwhile reading.

In almost any restaurant the artificial sweetener, provided on the tables, seems to be *Splenda*. The *nutrition facts* are printed on the reverse of the little package. The printing is so small it is difficult to read. Notwithstanding, an ingredient is *sucralose*—one of the sweeteners which featured in Professor Swithers' research, above. Another ingredient is *dextrose!* Dextrose is the equivalent of glucose and is derived from corn.

Amazingly, on the Splenda packet claims it to be a *no calorie sweetener.* But we know dextrose is assimilated immediately through the stomach walls and without delay increases the glucose or blood sugar levels. On the same packet is stated that this sweetener is 'suitable for people with diabetics.'

The short quote below; from an excellent article by Dr. David Brownstein titled *Avoid Artificial Sweeteners* (ref.39) and posted

September 3, 2012 should be enough to caution anyone on the hazards of artificial sweeteners:

"We are inundated with artificial sweeteners such as aspartame (Nutrasweet™) and sucralose (Splenda™). Nearly all of the low-fat food available is sweetened with an artificial sweetener. We have been told by the American Diabetes Association and the American Dietetic Association (now known as the Academy of Nutrition and Dietetics) that artificial sweeteners are a safe and effective way to lower caloric intake and help with weight loss. They are wrong.

Over the last 30 years, we have continually ingested more and more artificial sweeteners and there has been no decrease in our country-wide obesity problem. In fact, the opposite has occurred; as a population we are becoming more obese. Currently, two-thirds of Americans are overweight and one-third obese.

I have written extensively about artificial sweeteners in my newsletters and in my books. Artificial sweeteners do not help with weight loss. My experience has shown that, compared to those who do not ingest artificial sweeteners, those who ingest a large amount of artificial sweeteners tend to have more weight problems. Furthermore, it is much more difficult to lose weight when artificial sweeteners are ingested.

There are a whole host of problems associated with Nutrasweet™ ingestion including an increased risk for developing autoimmune and thyroid disorders, diabetes, obesity, and cancer. Splenda™ is no better. Animal studies of Splenda™ have shown it is associated with reduced growth rate in newborns, and adults, anemia, thyroid problems, mineral deficiencies (particularly magnesium) and various organ problems. Finally, never heat up an artificial sweetener or eat any product where an artificial sweetener has been added to a heated food or drink such as coffee. Heating Nutrasweet™ causes the chemical structure to change to a formaldehyde-like substance and Splenda™ can be converted into a dioxin-like molecule."

Before we move onto F.A.'s story below; it is worth recounting the brilliant work done and reported by Dr. Richard J. Johnson in his book *The Sugar Fix* (ref.8 p.xiv) in highlighting the dangers of fructose, and especially those of HFCS. It seems, from his research, the fructose causes an increase in uric acid—and that this compound in turn has an important influence on blood pressure. He states that diets rich in fructose appeared to be contributing to the growing obesity problem and rising rates of cardiovascular disease and other serious conditions.

F.A. recounted how he had been to his doctor for an annual check-up, and especially to obtain a detailed blood analysis. On his second visit, once the doctor had received the laboratory report, he was surprised when told his uric acid levels were dangerously high. In fact the doctor commented he was probably drinking too much wine—and what perturbed him was the uric acid would likely cause gout in the near future.

When he arrived home he shared his feelings of perplexity with his wife. They both knew he was only drinking two glasses of wine per week. F.A. said his wife *hit the nail on the head* when she reminded him he was eating about three slices of fruit cake a day. A cake loaded with raisins; and also containing sugar. She reasoned along these lines because wine is made from grapes, as are raisins.

We now know, from Dr. Johnson's work that F.A. was obtaining high levels of fructose both from the raisins and the sugar in the fruit cake.

Luckily, Dr. Johnson (ref.8 p.95) explains exactly what the uric acid does that causes the harm. It shuts down the production of nitric oxide which is necessary so the blood vessels can expand. When they cannot expand the pressure increases. In fact the uric acid is like a double edged sword because it *stimulates the production of angiotension which causes blood vessels to constrict.*

Much has been written on the health advantages of eating dark chocolate. However, IMO one needs to be careful and if partaking, to eat very small amounts. Be assured chocolate has to contain preservatives which are harmful; and in addition it contains sugar—and some chocolates now contain HFCS instead as it is cheaper, and extends the shelf-life. One needs to question whether the harm caused by these substances does not outweigh the benefits of the cocoa used to make dark chocolate. Additionally, some people find dark chocolate can cause headaches.

T.C. was a fellow who suddenly began getting rather severe headaches. They would occur late, every afternoon. One day he happened to mention this to his daughter who was away at residence in college, studying *home economics*. She responded by saying she did not know if it would help; but her lecturer had recently suggested that if a person was prone to headaches or migraine they should evaluate whether they were having too much of the 3C's—*coffee, cheese and chocolate!*

After his conversation with his daughter, T.C. said he had reflected on her comment and then realized he had begun eating cheese, three times a day, at about the time his headaches started. It was a yellow cheese that he had read would be good for health. However, to once again make a long story short—when he stopped eating the cheese, his headaches disappeared.

A.C. had a similar story to tell. He too would develop a frightening headache some afternoons—but only on certain weekdays. Eventually he pinpointed the problem as being a particularly delicious sandwich purchased for lunch at a restaurant near work. He said it had been loaded with a very yellow colored cheese.

K.D. was a young doctor who happened to be seated next to us on an airplane. During the flight the subject of headaches came up and he had an interesting story to tell. His father, who was also a doctor, had suffered terribly with headaches for a lengthy period of time—but only over the weekends. In the end they discovered the cause being that at his practice the father was drinking regular coffee: but at home his mother was using decaffeinated. It was the sudden caffeine withdrawal symptoms causing the headaches.

In his book, Alexander (ref.2 p.152) repeatedly warns about the hazards of eating acidic foods. Thus one should beware of anything sour—vinegar, lemon juice, grapefruit or grapefruit juice. And it is regarding the eating of acidic foods that makes J.S.'s story relatable:

J.S. was a lady who went on holiday with her family. At the place they stayed there was an abundance of tomatoes which were freely available. Consequently she had these at every meal. Then, she later told some friends, her arthritis in her hips suddenly flared up causing excruciating pain.

It would seem tomatoes are rather high in acid content, and as such destroys the essential oils in one's joints: hence the warning from Alexander, above, to avoid acidic or sour foods. Another warning comes from Margaret Durst (ref.18) and the following is a quote from one of her superb newsletters:

"One of the best and cheapest remedies is diet. Some basic arthritis causing or aggravating foods are peanuts, nightshades (potatoes, *tomatoes*, eggplant and peppers), soy, wheat, coffee and oranges. Food sensitivities can result in hidden inflammation—as in the kind that is in your joints and causes arthritis over time....... Diet changes can be as remarkable as any drug or supplement in eliminating joint pain and inflammation throughout the body.

Mineral deficiencies and imbalances contribute to arthritis as does an overly acid body pH. It is easy to test pH with litmus paper strips for urine. Anybody that is overly acid will have mineral imbalances that will start coming into harmony when pH is balanced."

Because vinegar is so acidic in nature a few comments regarding cider vinegar may be worthwhile.

B.A. was a fellow who told a group of acquaintances one evening about his problems with leg cramps the night before. He said he had been so desperate he resorted to drinking cider vinegar *neat and directly from the bottle.*

Curious as to how this could possibly have helped we checked out the label in the health store. On the bottle, under contents, it had written, "One tablespoon (15ml) contains 11mg potassium"—*nothing else was listed!*

We came to the conclusion the fellow obtained relief due to the potassium in the cider vinegar. This assessment was based on the work of Dr. Mercola (ref.17) and Sally Fallon (ref.11)—who state that leg cramps can result from a deficiency of potassium. What a terrible price the fellow was paying—short term relief because of the potassium; but with longer term harm in the joints from the vinegar.

S.W. was a retired engineer who wished to pass on to his nephew a secret formula for *staying healthy*. Simply it was a mixture, in equal parts, of cider vinegar and honey. He told his nephew he should take a tablespoon of this mixture each morning, which is what he personally had done all his life. Fortunately the nephew did not follow the advice, as today the uncle has arthritis severely in both knees.

As the above mixture contained half honey it is worth commenting that in his book Dr. Johnson (ref.8) warns of the hazards of honey: *as it is a super concentrated form of fructose.*

Then too there are some people who take honey before retiring at night. IMO people who take honey on an empty stomach before retiring at night are placing themselves in an extremely dangerous situation regarding blood sugar levels. The concentrated fructose will elevate the blood sugars and later, when the person is asleep, result in them *crashing below the two teaspoon* requirement level.

It was enlightening to read in Dr. Abrahamson's book (ref.3) how some people, who had been confined to hospital because of diabetes or hyperinsulinism; would be awakened during the night to be given a snack—as it was deemed necessary to maintain their sugar levels. One should never eat candy or drink alcohol immediately before retiring at night as this will definitely cause low blood sugars while asleep. It cannot be good for your body. And while we are not competent to talk about things like strokes one cannot help wondering how many occur during the early hours of the morning; and what was eaten—or not eaten—prior to going to sleep. Consequently, it may not do any harm to consider having a small protein type snack before retiring.

Genetically modified foods warrant a brief mention. For a deeper understanding of this subject we refer you to the doctors and authors in the References and Bibliography section of this book.

M.K. was a farmer who appeared on a TV News broadcast in Ireland at the turn of the century. He was being interviewed as part of a report on the "success" of genetically modified (GMO) maize, or corn as grown in the US. When the interviewer asked the farmer if his output of maize would increase when harvesting a crop coming from GMO seed he replied it definitely would saying, "Before I had to use insecticide to prevent the bugs from eating the maize. Now it's like the insecticide is inside the maize—because the bugs totally avoid it!"

Of course genetically modifying the corn has not *placed insecticide on the inside.* The farmer was speaking metaphorically to emphasize how "effective" the GMO crop was in repelling bugs.

It is worth repeating that the lower the form of life the more creatures are governed by inborn instinct—it is like *they are programmed.* Birds are born and soon after leaving the nest depart from their parents. When it is time for the new offspring to breed they are able to build nests for their young exactly as they should for their particular breed. Sea turtles hatch in the sea sand without having seen their mothers: yet they know to get into the ocean, what to eat and can return to where they were born 15 years later.

Bugs too know precisely what foods to eat without being shown by parents—in fact most bugs hatch and begin life never having seen their parents. But they instinctively know what to eat—*and what not to eat!*

Consequently, their 'built in instinct mechanism' cannot recognize the GMO corn or maize as food.

Just as miners in the early part of the last century used canaries in coalmines to determine if toxic gases were entering the mine shaft—so in a similar way the bug*s are warning you* this "new food" is not good for you. They are your *canary in the coalmine!*

Finally, because it is so harmful to health, a word on fluoride in drinking water: simply by providing two additional quotes (we have already quoted from Sally Fallon at the end of Chapter 1). The first from Wikipedia (ref.10):

"Arvid Carlsson, *winner of the 2000 Nobel Prize for Medicine,* opposes water fluoridation. He took part in the debate in Sweden, where he helped to convince Parliament that it should be illegal due to ethics. He believes that it violates modern pharmacological principles, which indicate that medications should be tailored to individuals.

Water fluoridation is still used in the United States, United Kingdom, Ireland, Canada, and Australia, and a handful of other countries. The following nations previously fluoridated their water [but then ceased the practice when the harmful effects were discovered]. Given in parentheses is the year of introduction; with the year it was stopped:

- Federal Republic of Germany (1952–1971)
- Sweden (1952–1971)
- Netherlands (1953–1976)
- Czechoslovakia (1955–1990)
- German Democratic Republic (1959–1990)
- Soviet Union (1960–1990)
- Finland (1959–1993)"

The final quote is from Dr. Mercola (ref.17):

"A recently published Harvard University meta-analysis funded by the National Institutes of Health (NIH) has concluded that children who live in areas with highly fluoridated water have *significantly lower* IQ scores than those who live in low fluoride areas."

Encouraging news is that in May, 2013, the citizens of Portland, Oregon, voted "No," thus rejecting the introduction of fluoride to their pristine drinking water supply.

What Is Good For You
—Chapter 21

When I was 16, I thought how little my
father knew. By the time I reached 21
—I was surprised at how much he
had learnt in the last five years.
                                    Mark Twain

The following list of *good-for-you-stuff* is by no means comprehensive. These tidbits are pieces of information uncovered during the research, and are presented with the view that what is good for overall general health is useful for arthritis.

Apples

Regarding apples, Refreshing News (ref.35) carried an attention-grabbing article in November, 2012 titled *An Apple a Day Keeps Cardiologists Away.* They were reporting on the work of lead researcher Robert DiSilvestro, professor of human nutrition at

Ohio State University and a researcher at the university's Ohio Agricultural Research and Development Center.

Professor DiSilvestro, reporting on a study funded by an apple industry group, found that apples lowered blood levels of oxidized LDL (low-density lipoprotein), the *"bad" cholesterol.*

According to the professor when LDL becomes oxidized, it takes on a form that begins atherosclerosis, or hardening of the arteries. From his study he found that people who ate one apple a day for four weeks have been found to have 40% lower blood levels of a substance linked to hardening of the arteries.

On another occasion Refreshing News (ref.35) had this to say about apples:

"One of the healthiest fruits you should be eating is one you probably already are: the apple. The Iowa Women's Health Study, which has been investigating the health habits of 34,000 women for nearly 20 years, named apples as one of only three foods (along with pears and red wine) that are most effective at reducing the risk of death from heart disease among postmenopausal women. Other massive studies have found the fruit [apples] lowers risk of lung cancer and type-2 diabetes—and even helps women lose weight. In fact, one of the only things that could make an apple unhealthy is *mixing it with sugar and flour*.....and stuffing it into a mile-high pie."

In the movie "The Gerson Miracle" (ref.28) it was stated that in his earlier life Dr. Gerson had suffered from migraine headaches. As a cure he devised a special diet and apples played a large part in what he subsequently ate.

However, it is useful to remember Dr. Johnson's findings in that one should be careful and not eat too much fructose. However, Dr. Johnson (Ref.8) also says eating dairy can negate some of the effects of sucrose. A suggestion, therefore, is sometimes to eat plain whole milk yogurt with diced raw apple, as it is delicious.

Broccoli

This comment regarding broccoli was found at Refreshing News (ref.35):

"Pick any life-threatening disease—cancer, heart disease, you name it—and eating more broccoli and its cruciferous cousins may help you beat it, Johns Hopkins research suggests. Averaging just four weekly servings of veggies like broccoli, cabbage, and cauliflower slashed the risk of dying from any disease by 26% among 6,100 people studied for 28 years."

Dr. Joseph Mercola (ref. 17) recently posted an informative article titled *Broccoli-Based Medicine—A Potent Tool Against Osteoarthritis and Cancer.* It will pay handsomely to access it and read the latest research on this powerful nourishing vegetable. Eating broccoli just has so many nutritional advantages!

Cabbage and Carrots

In their same article Refreshing News (ref.35) had these insights regarding cabbage and carrots:

"The humble cabbage is a thrifty cook's dream.....In spite of its low cost; it packs a nutritional punch, though. It's low in calories, but loaded with vitamins and minerals like Vitamins K and C, iron, calcium, and potassium."

"Carrots.....are excellent for you as they are high in vitamin A, thiamin, niacin, folate, vitamin B6, and a host of other nutrients."

Chicken Bones

Sally Fallon in *Nourishing Nutrition* (ref.11) has recommended the boiling of chicken bones and beef bones in a slow cooker, for a number of hours, to extract the calcium and other nutrients. So it was interesting to find these supporting comments at Chiropractic-help.com (ref.40):

"Harvard Medical School scientists report that a *chicken bones* extract is the source of a protein (gelatin)—and perhaps other substances—that *stopped the pain and swelling in a group* of 60 *rheumatoid arthritis patients who had not responded well to conventional medical treatment.*

Fermented Vegetables

Dr. Mercola (ref.17) writes extensively on the advantages of fermented vegetables, and how they improve the friendly gut bacteria. Similarly, here is a brief quote from Sally Fallon in *Nourishing Nutrition* (ref.11 p.97):

"A 1999 study published in the Lancet found that the consumption of lacto-fermented vegetables was positively associated with low rates of asthma, skin problems and autoimmune disorders in Swedish children attending a Waldorf school."

Garlic

Garlic has been referred to as *nature's antibiotic*. Accordingly, it seemed prudent to quote this comment from Refreshing News (ref.35):

"Garlic is a flavor essential and a health superstar in its own right. The onion relative contains more than 70 active phytochemicals, including allicin, which studies show may decrease high blood pressure by as much as 30 points. High consumption of garlic lowered rates of ovarian, colorectal, and other cancers, according to a research review in the *American Journal of Clinical Nutrition*. Allicin also fights infection and bacteria. British researchers gave 146 people either a placebo or a garlic extract for 12 weeks; garlic takers were two-thirds less likely to catch a cold."

Onions

Dale Alexander (ref.2) writes highly of the value of onions as a food. He also suggests that people suffering from constipation will find them useful in alleviating the condition.

Later, additional positive properties were found in Dr. van der Merwe's book *Health and Happiness* (ref.5 p.76) where she states that onions can reduce blood pressure and cholesterol. In addition they can prevent the formation of blood clots; as in thrombosis, heart attacks and stroke.

Protein

There is the characteristic that diets recommended for arthritics seem to contain generous amounts of protein, as has already been covered. The following are, therefore, merely additional quotes provided for information. The first is from Sally Fallon (ref.11 pp.26-27):

"When protein is lacking in the diet, there is a tendency for the blood and tissues to become either too acid or too alkaline, depending on the acidity or alkalinity of the foods we eat...... Just as animal fats are our only sources of vitamins A and D and other body building factors: so also animal protein is our only source of complete protein...... Protein cannot be adequately utilized without dietary fats. That is why protein and fats *occur together* in eggs, milk, fish and meat."

A word of caution here is that one must buy eggs high in omega-3 at the market or grocery store. Excess animal fats are included in the diet of hens these days which result in eggs low in omega-3 relative to omega-6. Similarly, while fat is essential in the diet as shown above—today with stall fed cattle, the content of the fat in the beef can be too high. Purchase grass fed beef if you are able.

On that note here is a quote from Refreshing News (ref.35) regarding lean beef:

"Lean beef is one of the best-absorbed sources of iron there is. (Too little iron can cause anemia.) Adding as little as 1 ounce of beef per day can make a big difference in the body's ability to absorb iron from other sources, says Mary J. Kretsch, PhD, a researcher at the USDA-ARS Western Human Nutrition Research Center in Davis, CA.

Beef also packs plenty of zinc (even minor deficiencies may impair memory) and B vitamins, which help your body turn food into energy. If you can, then splurge on grass fed beef. Compared with grain fed beef, it has twice the concentration of vitamin E, a powerful brain boosting antioxidant. It's also high in omega-3 fatty acids. Because this type of beef tends to be lower in overall fat, it can be tough—so marinate it, and use a meat thermometer to avoid overcooking."

Finally, in his book *Wheat Belly* Dr. W. Davis (ref.9 p.208) recommends one should eat *meat and eggs.*

Potassium Foods

Dr. Mercola has written about the advantages of potassium bearing foods: as a means of balancing the potassium to salt ratio in the diet; and in explaining how essential it is for attaining overall health.

To obtain a list of those foods high in potassium you can search on Google, or access Dr. Mercola's website (ref.17).

Dr. Richard J. Johnson (ref.8 p.252) also gives an inventory of potassium rich foods from which he recommends frequent servings.

Refreshing News (ref.35) later carried a similar article on the necessity of this mineral in the diet. In their excellent write up they reported that in a recent 5-year study from the Netherlands, high potassium diets were linked with lower rates of death from all causes in healthy adults age 55 and older.

Here is a partial list of foods containing potassium: asparagus; avocados; beans (legumes, dried beans, especially lima beans); milk; mushrooms; nuts; potatoes and sweet potatoes; pumpkin and winter squash

Finally, while discussing the diet of the 100 year old man, who had recovered from terminal cancer in the story titled *The Island Where People Forgot To Die* (ref.7), and as discussed in Chapter 11; Dan Buettner mentions that the inhabitants of the area always included beans and homegrown potatoes in their lunch menu. *Both are rich in potassium.*

Raw Versus Roasted Nuts

At one stage during the research we were at a loss whether we should purchase raw or roasted nuts to obtain the maximum nutritional benefit. Then we discovered that a potential hazard to purchasing cooked or roasted nuts is that hydrogenated oils may have been used in the process. To be healthy necessitates avoiding such oils—which are used as a preservative. Consequently, we only purchased raw nuts.

Regarding eating raw nuts Dr. W. Davis (ref.9 p.207) states they are filling and full of fiber, monounsaturated oils, and protein. Additionally, they reduce blood pressure and LDL cholesterol. He does caution though, that peanuts are not nuts, but legumes and should not be consumed raw. Most encouragingly he claims that consuming raw nuts several times a week can *add two years to your life!*

Dr. Richard J. Johnson (ref.8 p.265) is also a proponent of eating nuts and says that lentils and nuts (especially hazelnuts, walnuts and peanuts), are excellent sources of the amino acid, L-arginine.

Red Wine

On this subject, Dr. Richard J. Johnson (ref.8 p.185) claims drinking red wine each day is good for you. He says small servings of wine will help to lower the risk of cardiovascular disease by raising levels of HDL cholesterol—the *good* kind. The reason being that red wine contains an antioxidant known as resveratrol which increases production of nitric oxide. And as previously mentioned this compound helps your blood vessels.

Salads

Growing up as a child you might remember salads being placed on the lunch and dinner table. From Sally Fallon (ref.11 p.95) we read that consuming raw uncooked food along with a meal *can take the load off* the pancreas. She quotes from Dr. Edward Howell's book *Food Enzymes for Health and Longevity* when she states:

"A certain amount of raw, uncooked food in the diet *is indispensible* to the highest degree of health."

Sardines

Sardines are mentioned by Alexander (ref.2) as a good source of omega-3 oils for arthritis. They are inexpensive, and with the controversy surrounding the ill effects of farmed salmon; and with wild salmon being so expensive—they are a good source of these oils. Refreshing News (ref.35) has this comment:

"Like many fish, sardines [canned] are high in healthy omega-3 fatty acids, but unlike many larger fish, they are low in mercury and PCBs. That makes them a wonderful choice, especially for women who are pregnant or nursing. Even better, they can be eaten straight from the tin, or cooked, added to a sauce, or almost anything else you can think of, and are one of the most affordable fishes on the market."

Spinach

All vegetables are essential, but it is worth reviewing these enlightening comments from Refreshing News (ref.35):

"Spinach.…..contains lots of lutein, the sunshine-yellow pigment found in egg yolks. Aside from guarding against age-related macular degeneration, a leading cause of blindness, lutein may prevent heart attacks by keeping artery walls clear of cholesterol.

Spinach is also rich in iron, which helps deliver oxygen to your cells for energy, and folate, a B vitamin that prevents birth defects. Cook frozen spinach leaves (they provide more iron when cooked than raw) and serve as a side dish with dinner a few times a week."

Sweet Potatoes

Much has been written of the value of sweet potatoes. One can eat them without the weight gaining effect of ordinary potatoes according to Mark Sisson (ref.6). This quote is from Refreshing News (ref.35) when they recently wrote on the subject of sweet potatoes:

"One of the best ways to get vitamin A—an essential nutrient that protects and maintains eyes, skin, and the linings of our respiratory, urinary, and intestinal tracts—is from foods containing beta-carotene, which your body converts into the vitamin. Beta carotene-rich foods include carrots, squash, kale, and cantaloupe, but sweet potatoes have among the most. A half-cup serving of these sweet spuds delivers only 130 calories but 80 percent of the daily value of vitamin A."

Sunlight

The more we research the more it is apparent how essential it is to get, as an absolute minimum, at least 10 minutes of direct sunshine each day. Some commentators would argue you need more. When your body is exposed to the sunlight it manufactures vitamin D in the skin. This vitamin is required for the absorption of calcium.

Other benefits are that exposure to sunlight affects one's mood for the better: and surprisingly helps with a better night's sleep. A suggestion is to combine your time in the sun with some exercise such as walking or bicycle riding. When you think about it we were not designed to be indoors most of the time.

Dr. Mercola (ref.17) posted an informative *must-read* article on the benefits of sunlight. Here is a small quote:

"In fact, exposure to the sun may be one of the most important steps you can take in preventing heart disease and stroke. Scientists at the University of Edinburgh discovered that when sunlight touches your skin, *nitric oxide is released into your bloodstream* and nitric oxide is a powerful blood pressure lowering compound."

Yogurt

A pleasant and nutritious way of improving gut bacteria is through eating yogurt.

Some good news is that *"Dannon all natural, plain yogurt"* is preservative free! It is made from whole milk: and while the milk may have been pasteurized it does not seem to have been homogenized. It contains the good bacteria, acidophilus; along with other bacteria. It also contains many vitamins and minerals which are listed on the container.

Another benefit of eating yogurt is from Sally Fallon in *Nourishing Nutrition* (ref.11 p.33):

"The practice of fermenting or souring milk is found in almost all traditional groups that keep herds. This process partially breaks down lactose and predigests casein. Yoghurt and kefir are well tolerated by adults who cannot drink fresh milk."

Vitamins And Supplements
—Chapter 22

**A little knowledge
is a dangerous thing**
American Proverb

The deeper we delve into this subject, the greater our perception of how little we know! And of how much there is to learn on the subject of vitamins and supplements. For example, who would have thought that in taking one type of vitamin; one can actually cause a shortage of another? To make matters much worse—the manufacturers of vitamins do not place warnings to this fact on the bottles of their product.

Many folk do not *believe in* vitamins—possibly to their detriment. Rightly, they say they should be in the food we eat. But modern farming methods can deplete the soils of certain necessary nutrients, plus delays from time of harvesting to time of consumption can result in the deterioration of vitamin content. In addition modern processing methods can completely denude certain foodstuffs of their vitamin content.

However, while vitamins and nutrients are essential—the way to take them, to achieve maximum benefit for the body, may be in limited quantities: and only after research into the side effects as well as the potential benefits of the type you are considering taking. One should never take them 'willy-nilly' and in no way exceed recommended doses.

An Introduction

We learn about vitamins when some kind person tells or educates us, or via shared personal learning situations. If the stories told are authentic and interesting they lead to an understanding of the importance of these nutrients in the diet. Here are a few such learning situations:

B.K. was a teacher in middle school. He had a beautiful knack of making his lectures both fascinating and informative, and the way he did this was to tell his students of real life experiences from time to time.

On one occasion he told the story of how the English and Americans, immediately following the Second World War, and while they had a presence in the Far East; had introduced refined rice to the local population. Now these people had traditionally eaten the brown whole rice, and were amazingly healthy. But because the new white rice was tastier (sweeter) and easier to prepare it was readily accepted.

However, after a time, the administrators noticed there was an alarming increase in the number of cases of beriberi. They called in their doctors and scientists who discovered that the beriberi was occurring because of a shortage of the B vitamins in the new diet. They also found this shortage had come about because the B vitamins were in the brown bran covering the rice—and which the people were no longer eating since the advent of the refined product.

Subsequently, the English and Americans devised ways to extract the B vitamins from the bran—and then sold these vitamins to the local people to cure their beriberi infections.

B.K. taught his class about vitamins on another occasion. This opportunity came about when studying the early Portuguese explorers, such as Vasco da Gama. This seafaring captain, and his compatriots, had opened a route to the Far East in the 15th century (round the Cape of Good Hope on the most southern part of the African continent) in order to obtain spices for Europe.

Because of the long voyage and the perishable nature of vegetables many of the sailors would develop scurvy from a lack of vitamin C. Consequently a refitting station had to be set up in what is now Cape Town in South Africa. While giving these facts B.K. had gone on to explain about vitamin C and which fruits and vegetables contained the vitamin. It was a golden opportunity to introduce his class to the essential nature of vitamins.

S.B. was another teacher, also in middle school, and although it was not part of the curriculum, she had her students compile charts of the different vegetables; and then to list under each the vitamins and nutrients they contained: such as iron and zinc. The students found the subject fascinating and would go home and share with their parents what they had learnt that day.

In this way these two teachers taught their students an early appreciation of the nutritious advantages of eating healthy foods.

I.C. was a fellow who suffered continually with fibrositis. The spasms of muscle cramps and pain in his shoulders were often so severe that his wife would need to massage his back before he could get any sleep at night.

Then, as it chanced they went on safari to a wild nature reserve in Africa. Because their arrival was in the middle of summer, and as it was in a malaria area for that time of year: they had to take anti-malaria pills. Now, the contra-indications on the leaflet which came with the pills stated that the medication could cause a folic acid (a B vitamin) shortage; and recommended it be taken simultaneously—which they did.

They had a fantastic vacation, and the thing that helped was the fact that I.C. did not experience any of the normal discomfort due to fibrositis.

When, not too long after his return home—and the pain had started up again—his wife made the comment that he had not experienced any fibrositis while taking the folic acid, while on vacation. Consequently, she had wondered if the folic acid could perhaps be a cure for the fibrositis.

To make a long happy story short: I.C. went and bought some folic acid and noticed that once again the pain disappeared. He told us that since the discovery, he had continued taking folic acid and as a result has hardly ever experienced the pain associated with fibrositis. And that if ever it did recur, then all he needed to do, for a brief period, was to increase the amount taken.

I.C. had another story to share. On this occasion it had a happy outcome as well: due to a relative giving him Dr. van der Merwe's book *Health and Happiness* (ref.5).

For many years he had suffered from vertigo (dizziness) which had occurred about every six months. On those occasions it would be so bad he had to stay in bed for about three days until it cleared up. It became particularly embarrassing when the fellows at work suggested it was a result of stress, thus implying his job position was too demanding.

Regrettably, the frequency of the *attacks* began increasing until eventually they were occurring every six weeks—all requiring bed rest. Without the medication which his doctor had prescribed he did not know how he would have managed. As time went on the vertigo turned into Meniere's disease, and his hearing began becoming impaired.

Finally, during one particularly bad attack, his wife said she was going to look through Dr. van der Merwe's book, which they had recently received, to see if it contained a suggested remedy. And true enough—it stated the ailment was the result of a shortage of vitamin B3 (niacin).

As if *by magic*—the niacin really worked! The fellow says it was so comforting to finally find a cure for his problem, and to have done so by tackling the actual cause!

Pungent Facts

Vitamin A

In her book *Nourishing Nutrition* (ref.11 p.37) Sally Fallon refers to the work of Dr. Price. Here is the particular quote:

"According to Dr. Price, protein, minerals and water-soluble vitamins cannot be utilized by the body without vitamin A from animal sources.....Sources include egg yolks, liver and organic meats, seafood and fish liver oils."

Vitamin B Complex

The B vitamins are essential to health. The few stories above illustrate this adequately. What makes the 'shortage situation' worse is that our traditional sources for these vitamins and supplements have been denied us with the advent of GMO wheat and corn. Therefore, we must now seek alternative foods containing these vitamins to remain healthy.

Before providing a brief summary of the well known types of B vitamins, it may be appropriate to add this fact: Vitamin B3 or niacin is useful in overcoming stress and a whole bunch of disorders: for example Meniere's disease as in the story above. However, if one takes too much it can cause a shortage of lecithin. And if you were to take lecithin it could affect your system's ability to absorb calcium, because of the phosphorous content.

Just another reason why you should be wary; and not exceed recommended doses.

This abridged summary of the B vitamins was obtained from Margaret Durst (ref.18) and is as follows:

"B vitamins are also produced by the healthy bacteria in the intestinal tract. The B vitamins are known for promoting proper functioning of the brain and nervous system. They help bring relaxation and energy to those who are stressed out and fatigued. B vitamins are also important to the health of the skin, hair, eyes and liver. B vitamins (taken in the day) are also one of my favorite remedies for insomnia.

Vitamin B1 or thiamine is essential for proper digestion and nerve function. Major indicators of deficiency include irritability, depression, apathy, and burning or tingling in the soles of the feet.

B2 is also known as riboflavin. It is important for energy. Symptoms of deficiency include eye problems, bloodshot eyes, cracks in the corners of the mouth, and dermatitis.

B3 is niacin. Niacin helps lower cholesterol and improves blood flow through the capillaries. Extreme redness and roughness of the skin is one of the first signs of niacin deficiency. Other symptoms of deficiency include canker sores, indigestion, weakness, memory loss and anxiety.

B5 is pantothenic acid and is closely associated with the function of the adrenal cortex. Symptoms of deficiency include fatigue, hypoglycemia, and increased allergy symptoms.

B6 is pyridoxine. B6 has a multitude of functions. It is especially important in the function of the central nervous system.

Symptoms of deficiency include tremors, skin diseases, carpal tunnel syndrome, motion sickness, tendency towards fainting and arteriosclerosis. B6 is also very helpful in women for symptoms of fluctuating hormone levels.

Folic acid is B9. It is very closely linked to B12 or cobalamin. Both are important to energy and an overall feeling of wellbeing. Symptoms of deficiency include anemia, fatigue, general weakness, nerve problems and difficulty with muscular coordination."

In her book Dr. van der Merwe (ref.5 p.145, p.213) states that taking 100mg/day of choline along with inositol is beneficial as it forms part of acetylcholine. This compound is essential for memory, learning ability and intellectual alertness. In addition taking 100mg/day of inositol helps the nervous system and also helps with insomnia.

She also maintains that taking 100mgm/day of vitamin B12, or cobalamin, will increase energy levels and improve the activity of the nervous system. It is known as the energy and longevity vitamin and is used in the treatment of fatigue; depression; insomnia; anxiety; poor memory; osteoporosis *and arthritis.*

Vitamin C

Dr. Richard J. Johnson (Ref.8 p.251) recommends taking vitamin C, as plain ascorbic acid, on a daily basis. His advice is to take 250 mg per day as greater amounts may cause kidney stones. He makes this recommendation because he has found that people who have high blood pressure and heart disease also tend to have low blood levels of vitamin C. Additionally vitamin C appears to offset some of fructose's damaging effects.

Adelle Davis (ref.4) writes extensively on how essential vitamin C is to health. She has a whole chapter on its values and gives case studies of how arthritis was successfully treated with large doses of this vitamin. However, from our research, one should always take vitamin C with a meal and not on an empty stomach.

Doctor van der Merwe (ref.5 p.129) informs us that vitamin C ensures that calcium is absorbed into the osteoblasts. These are the bone cells that are responsible for the formation of bone and the deposits of calcium in the bone. Therefore, she suggests taking about 200mg of vitamin C in the evenings along with your calcium and magnesium to aid absorption.

She goes on to say that vitamin C also plays a role in the relief of backache pain, caused by slipped discs—*and all inflammatory pain associated with arthritis.*

Refreshing News (ref.35) supports this claim regarding arthritis when they recount how Australian scientists recently discovered that vitamin C reduces knee pain *by protecting your knees against arthritis.* Furthermore, Finnish researchers found that men with low levels of the vitamin were 2.4 times likelier to have a stroke.

This final quote is from Wikipedia, the free encyclopedia (ref.10):

"Vitamin C or L-ascorbic acid.... is an essential nutrient for humans and certain other animal species......Deficiency in this vitamin causes the disease scurvy in humans. Ascorbic acid is also widely used as a food additive, to prevent oxidation."

Vitamin D

Adelle Davis (ref.4 p.121) has this to say regarding this essential vitamin:

"Vitamin D can be absorbed into the blood only in the presence of fat. A great increase in rickets has been reported in both the United States and Canada because physicians, untrained in nutrition, recommend that infants and children be given skim milk."

According to Adelle Davis (ref.4 p.121) one of the better means of obtaining vitamin D is through taking fish-liver oils. She describes the case of a two year old child whom she treated and who was cured of rickets by being given:

"Two teaspoons of cod-liver oil daily for a year and a teaspoonful daily since and has now become a beautifully formed, handsome boy."

In reading this quote from Adelle Davis it is important to recall her research was done in the 1970's and the cod liver oil was from that time; and was possibly less concentrated than those available today.

Sally Fallon in *Nourishing Nutrition* (ref.11 p.39) gives the benefits of taking vitamin D, and also warns of the danger of synthetic vitamin D2. She writes:

"The body manufactures vitamin D3 out of cholesterol in the presence of sunlight.....Dr. Price found that healthy primitive diets were rich in vitamin D foods like eggs, liver, organ meats, marine oils and seafood..... *Synthetic D2 has been linked to hyperactivity, coronary heart disease and other allergic reactions.*"

Vitamin D is essential for the absorption of calcium. The healthiest way to obtain your vitamin D is from sunlight. Sunburn is the body's built in safety mechanism so you do not take in, or rather manufacture too much. That said it seems the minimum requirement is at least 10 minutes in the sun each day. Then there are other benefits from exposure to sunlight such as a happier disposition along with better sleep at night, etc. If you access Dr. Mercola (ref.17) you will find he has written extensively on the subject.

As previously stated, cod liver oil also supplies you with this essential vitamin.

In some instances it is unavoidable taking synthetic vitamin D3 as manufacturers' combine it with calcium in their supplements. If you do take these supplements keep an eye out as to the total amount of vitamin D consumed in a day; as excessive amounts may be harmful.

Vitamin E

Adelle Davis (ref.4 p.139) goes to great lengths to stress the importance of vitamin E. The following quote is provided because we have recommend taking oils including cod liver oil; and because she cautions there is an increased need for vitamin E when taking these oils:

"The amount of vitamin E needed daily varies widely....The need is increased by stress, the intake of oils, long deprivation of this vitamin....because a small increase in the intake of oils, or unsaturated fats, can increase the need for vitamin E six fold, it is extremely dangerous to add oils to the diet without simultaneously obtaining more vitamin E."

With reference to the amount of vitamin E one should take when oils are increased in the diet, Adelle Davis (ref.4 p.139) gives these guidelines:

"Estimates of the daily requirement [of vitamin E] run from a bare minimum of 30 units to several hundred units. Careful studies indicate that an adult usually needs 140 to 210 units' daily but requires 100 additional units for each tablespoon of oil in the diet. A small excess is stored in the pituitary, adrenal and sex glands, but it is quickly exhausted, especially during illness. The amounts which have produced excellent results have usually been 600 to 1,600 units daily, always taken after meals containing fat.

Persons who have uncontrolled high blood pressure or hearts damaged from chronic rheumatic fever, however, should take no more than 100 units of vitamin E daily for the first six weeks.....The amount can then be increased to 125 units daily and six weeks later to 150 units."

Calcium

Today's diet can be sorely lacking in calcium and supplements may be a good idea. However, if you take them do not exceed 1,200mg calcium per day. IMO calcium citrate is best for absorption.

One should also be aware that taking calcium on its own can cause a magnesium shortage. They are normally taken in the ratio of two parts calcium to one part magnesium, i.e. 600mg magnesium balances 1,200mg calcium.

That said here are some comments from people who know. The first is from Adelle Davis (ref.4 p.145):

"Before calcium can pass through the intestinal wall into the blood it must first be dissolved by hydrochloric acid in the stomach. If the diet is excessively high in phosphorus, calcium and phosphorus combine in the intestine to make insoluble salts which do not dissolve even in acid. *Concentrated carbohydrate stimulates the flow of alkaline digestive juices, which decreases or prevents the absorption of calcium.*

The last sentence in her quote refers specifically to sugars, and refined carbohydrates. Then, regarding her comment on the hazards of too much phosphorus in the diet; is what makes one think twice before taking lecithin as a supplement because of its high phosphorus content.

The next quote is from Sally Fallon (ref.11 p.41):

"Best sources of calcium are dairy products and bone broth......Excess magnesium can inhibit calcium absorption, as can phosphorus, iron and zinc......Sugar consumption and stress both pull calcium from the bones."

You did note that additional hazard regarding eating sugar from Sally Fallon, above? It seems there is no end to the harm it causes.

Magnesium

Magnesium has to be about the most essential mineral supplement one can take. A shortage can cause *depression and crabbiness,* in addition to listlessness and a feeling of exhaustion. Some health professionals have written about the difficulties associated with the body's ability to absorb magnesium. And different authors recommend diverse types such as magnesium sulphate, magnesium chloride, magnesium oxide or magnesium citrate.

It is probably a *preference thing,* but our first choice is magnesium oxide as we have found it is best for absorption and produces the best results.

Sally Fallon (ref.11 p.42) has penned this comment regarding magnesium:

"Magnesium deficiency can result in: coronary heart disease, chronic weight loss, obesity, fatigue, epilepsy and impaired brain function......A diet high in carbohydrates can cause deficiencies."

Then Dr. van der Merwe (ref.5 p.127), who has written so extensively on supplements, says that low magnesium levels can result in slow digestion of food and increased irritability: along with tremor, muscle spasm, muscle cramps, muscle strain and facial tics.

Zinc

Because of modern farming methods together with the widespread use of fertilizers; foods today are lacking in adequate quantities of this important mineral. One can verify this statement by pointing to the large proportion of men who suffer from enlarged or benign prostrate in their later years as they get older. Some figures suggest the number of men suffering with this problem exceeds 50 percent. We suspect, of course, that refined carbohydrates have exacerbated the problem.

However, the good news is that merely by taking a zinc supplement each day it will definitely alleviate the problem.

Though, a word of caution regarding taking zinc—as large amounts of zinc will cause a copper shortage. Therefore, you will need to take a copper supplement as well.

Iodine

Because her comment is relevant this quote from Sally Fallon (ref.11 p.44) is included here:

"Germanium rich foods *help combat rheumatoid arthritis* – [and are] found in garlic, ginseng, mushrooms, onions… if present in the soil…..Although needed in only minute amounts, *iodine* is essential for…fat metabolism, thyroid function and the production of sex hormones…..Signs of deficiency are: proneness to weight gain, poor memory, constipation, depression and headaches…..*In excess iodine can be toxic.*"

Potassium

We have resisted taking potassium supplements; preferring instead to get potassium from those foods rich in them. This is easy enough to do and has definite health benefits besides. Dr. Mercola (ref.17) recommends getting your potassium through diet and has given a comprehensive list of these foods that includes things like lima and pinto beans as well as broccoli.

Dr. Richard J. Johnson (ref.8 p.252) gives a pertinent warning about taking potassium supplements when he says that high blood levels of potassium can cause cardiac arrest, especially in people with kidney disease. Therefore, one should not take them unless your doctor tells you to.

Unpleasant Experiences
—Chapter 23

**Whom the Gods would destroy
they first make crazy.**
German Proverb

B.J. was a semi-retired man who had received a visit from a relative. Now this relative had been suffering, and struggling greatly for some time with arthritis. He had over the years tried various medications to help relieve the pain. Knowing his experience, B.J. asked his advice about the 'cricking' he was beginning to experience in his knees: to which the relative most strongly suggested he take *glucosamine chondroitin*. He maintained it was the perfect thing to nourish the knee joints.

Consequently, B.J. went out and purchased a supply, and began taking it as prescribed. But after a few days he began to feel a bit of backache and thought nothing of it other than maybe he had slightly overextended a muscle or something. However, by the end of the first week of taking the glucosamine chondroitin, the backache was so severe he could hardly walk.

It got so bad it began to affect his sleep; and lying in bed early one morning, he began to mull over what changes he had made to his diet that could possibly have caused the pain he was suffering. Suddenly, in an instant he remembered he had introduced the glucosamine chondroitin to his regnum. To determine if it was the culprit he immediately ceased taking the stuff—and after one week his back pain had gone.

In telling the story he mentioned it was really lucky the pain had happened so soon after he commenced taking the medication—or he might not have recognized the cause of it. Summing up he said he did not know if the product was directly to blame or whether some additive or preservative had been added by the manufacturer; to the particular brand he had purchased.

Researching glucosamine chondroitin on Google, we chanced upon a website QuackWatch.org (ref.41), with comments from Dr. Stephen Barrett. Here are some brief quotes from his excellent article:

"Glucosamine supplements are derived from shellfish shells; chondroitin supplements are generally made from cow cartilage….. Chondroitin appears to be useless. Whether glucosamine is useful is conflicting….. [The] bottom line….. *Benefit is unlikely.*"

After hearing B.J.'s story and reading Dr. Barrett's full article it seems especially wise and prudent to keep away from glucosamine chondroitin supplements.

Now R.P. was a fellow who believed in taking vitamin and mineral supplements. Then at one stage he read that vitamin C can be more readily absorbed if the manufacturer had added flavonoids to the product. So he went and purchased a brand packaged by a renowned food store chain.

After about six months he developed the most intense itch, all over his body and especially on his legs, which occurred mainly at night. It was so bad he would be awakened from his sleep with the itch. Unbelievably this suffering continued for over a year before he established the cause.

He says that what made detecting the cause so difficult was that at first he was told certain foods such as granny smith apples, or raisins would cause such itching—and so began a process of cutting out certain foods to determine the offender: but all to no avail.

When nothing was discovered in his food source he eventually turned to the vitamins and supplements he was taking, eliminating them one at a time and watching for signs of improvement. And it was only when the least suspected—the vitamin C—was eliminated from the diet; did the itchy rash disappear.

A word of caution can be added in that some flavonoids are made from the peel of lemons—and we now know how acidic that may be. Therefore, the advice from Dr. Richard J. Johnson (ref.8) seems best—for vitamin C, stick to plain ascorbic acid.

In a similar situation, T.S. was a teenager who had been told that the way to maintain perfect health was to eat a wedge of pure baking yeast each day. As the years rolled by he could not understand his loss of hair—so much so that by the time he reached his early 20's he was bald. It was years later, while reading one of Adelle Davis' books, when the riddle was solved. She explicitly stated that eating raw baking yeast would cause one's hair to fall out.

Then too, there was the situation K.R. found himself in. He and his wife had moved to Ireland for a spell. While there he did everything he could to eat naturally; avoiding all refined and processed foods and those containing preservatives—so he was mystified when he began getting migraine headaches. Then one day by chance he happened to hear news broadcast on TV, which stated that, although Ireland had a largely agricultural economy; the chain stores had been importing a large amount of beef from Spain.

The news commentator had then gone on to say that the beef in question was found to be causing migraine headaches amongst consumers. It seemed that the beef producers in Spain had been injecting their cattle with growth hormones to maximize profits. And the reason for the migraines was due to these hormones in the beef. Once again, the relevance of this story is that there *always* has to be a cause!

Then there are simply *bad vitamins*. Consider M.T.'s story:

M.T. had been told not to *buy cheap* when purchasing his supply of vitamin B complex—so he bought an expensive brand. Then after nine months, or so, he began to develop 'pins and needles' in his upper left arm.

At that time he was spending a large amount of time in front of his laptop as it provided his income. So he thought it had to be posture and sought to ensure he had the correct chair with the right height for his work station, and so on. When this did not help he surmised it might be due to a lack of exercise, and increased his efforts at getting fit.

When none of these helped he began eliminating, slowly and one at a time, the vitamin supplements he was using. Little did he suspect it could be his B complex; so left these until last. Finally, however, he got around to deleting them from his regnum and after awhile began to feel a remarkable improvement. It did, though, take a full month for his arm to return to normal.

He said what had made it so difficult to detect the real culprit was the length of time it took before he noticed the onset of the problem—and he wondered if perhaps he had to get a 'build-up' in his system first?

Later we uncovered an article on Lewrockwell.com, which had been written by Daisy Luther and originally posted on the TheOrganicPrepper.ca (ref.1). It was titled *10 Ways to Commit Nutritional Anarchy* and reported on some abuses adopted in the retail of vitamins. This short extract is provided for information:

"Once upon a time, if we felt we needed to, we could go to the pharmacy or department store, select a bottle of vitamins, and feel pretty confident about the actual contents of the bottles.

Nowadays, real vitamins are so hard to track down that they might as well be on the endangered species list.

In fact, most of what is sold as "vitamins" in the United States actually contains toxic ingredients and nutritional content that isn't readily bio-available. And matters may soon get even worse, as the US government "harmonizes" with an overbearing set of rules called Codex Alimentarius.

Just going to the drug-store and buying one of the brightly colored bottles off the shelf may actually be worse for your health than being bereft of the nutrient. Before spending your hard-earned money on candy flavored chewables or much-advertised over-the-counter vitamin imposters, do some research. Recently, Sayer Ji of Green Med Info wrote about the hazardous chemicals found in a popular brand of children's vitamins:

"Kids vitamins are supposed to be healthy, right? Well then, what's going on with **Flintstones Vitamins**, which proudly claims to be "Pediatricians' #1 Choice"? Produced by the global pharmaceutical corporation Bayer, this wildly successful brand features a shocking list of unhealthy ingredients, including:

"Aspartame, Cupric Oxide, Coal tar artificial coloring agents (FD&C Blue #2, Red #40, Yellow #6), Zinc Oxide, Sorbitol, Ferrous Fumarate, Hydrogenated Oil (Soybean) and GMO Corn starch."

On Bayer Health Science's Flintstones product page designed for healthcare professionals they lead into the product description with the following tidbit of information:

"82% of kids aren't eating all of their veggies (1). Without enough vegetables, kids may not be getting all of the nutrients they need."

The implication—those Flintstones vitamins somehow fill this nutritional void.

With the approach of a world governed by Codex Alimentarius, natural supplements will become regulated to the point that you will no longer be able to acquire a therapeutic amount without taking nutritionally pillaged vitamins by the handful.

In the United States, the FDA is in charge of implementing the standards. Over the next two years, with the Food Safety Modernization Act, they will be doing just that. According to a Natural News article by Dr. Gregory D'Amato, these irrevocable standards are on their way to being implemented to allow the US to "harmonize" with Codex.

* All nutrients (vitamins and minerals) are to be considered toxins/poisons and are to be removed from all food because Codex prohibits the use of nutrients to "prevent, treat or cure any condition or disease"

* All nutrients (e.g., CoQ10, Vitamins A, B, C, D, Zinc and Magnesium) that have any positive health impact on the body will be deemed illegal under Codex and are to be reduced to amounts negligible to humans' health.

Basically what it all boils down to is that we have to be responsible for ourselves, to get the nutrients we need. Soon legitimate vitamins will not be readily available—only the toxic Big Pharma options will be sold. Because of this, it is imperative that we figure out how to provide these things for ourselves.

One article suggests that once Codex is fully implemented, most vitamins and nutritional supplements will require a prescription. Drug companies can exploit this process by trying to patent common dietary ingredients as drugs, before supplement companies have an opportunity to submit their NDI notifications. Once a drug company investigates an ingredient for drug purposes and publishes their findings, the ingredient can no longer be used in supplements."

Daisy Luther (ref.1) has some pertinent and useful information and ideas on how to become self-sufficient nutrient and vitamin wise. Therefore, visiting her site and reviewing her full article of July 26, 2013 will be worth your while.

Assessment of Chapters 22 and 23

If you can improve, or regain, your health by taking certain nutrients and vitamins then surely this is the thing to do? For example, if you have vertigo, or some serious disability such as multiple sclerosis, your first approach should be to see what Dr. van der Merwe suggests in her book (ref.5); or read up on the websites listed in the *References* section. This is a suggested best approach before starting some medication which might well cause some unpleasant and debilitating side effect.

While on the subject, and concerning multiple sclerosis, Dr. van der Merwe has so much sound advice that can only help. She recommends taking vitamin E and selenium; and illustrates how essential magnesium and calcium are—and not only for the multiple sclerosis sufferer; but for the arthritic as well. Her knowledge of the B vitamins is weighty and essential reading for the sufferer.

Only do your research, and keep your journal up to date so as to guard against those supplements containing stuff that may disagree with you. When you discover, through trial and error what works best for you, try and limit your intake. The last thing one would want to become is a *pill popper* with all sorts of vitamins and supplements in the cupboard.

One's first line of approach should be to always eat healthy wholesome and nourishing foods.

Finally though, we can testify to the personal health benefits from sound nutrient and vitamin supplements: and have witnessed these improvements in others.

Saving You Money
—Chapter 24

Questioning is the door to knowledge.

Anon

Eating healthy food saves you money even while you are sleeping! Just think of the savings in keeping out of hospitals; away from doctors and avoiding those awful expensive medications.

During a discussion on the topic of eating nourishing food, W.K. told his colleagues at work of an incident from his childhood.

He said that a friend, whose parents were exceedingly wealthy, had become ill. What he remembered most about his friend being taken to visit a doctor; was the outrage and indignation of the mother. It came about when the doctor diagnosed her son as being malnourished. The woman seemingly took this as inferred criticism that she did not know how to feed her family.

W.K. said the real problem had been that with their wealth they had overindulged in all the "good things" like candy and ice-cream, etc. In his book *Sugar Blues* (ref.20), William Dufty tells of how, when sugar was initially introduced to England, it was so expensive that only the wealthy could afford to eat things like chocolate regularly. So they were the ones who developed diabetes.

One needs to dispel the myth that to eat healthily one has to spend a fortune. Rather, it simply means knowing how to shop and how to plan meals: to minimize the work involved. For example, when preparing a meal make it large enough for two sittings. Eat the first portion on the day prepared and refrigerate the remainder until the next day.

If planning to eat oats for breakfast one can soak them in water overnight so they will cook in three minutes the following morning. Similarly soaking beans overnight shortens the cooking time next day—and saves on electricity.

Other savings can be made by using a slow cooker to make bone broth, as was described by Sally Fallon in *Nourishing Nutrition* (ref.11 p.29):

"Individuals who must restrict protein consumption for budgetary reasons: should include liberal amounts of good quality animal fats and budget-sparing bone broth in their diets."

Returning to the savings from dried beans this quote from Refreshing News (ref.35) is valuable:

"Protein is often the most expensive element of a meal, but beans are one of the rare exceptions. You can usually buy a one pound bag for a dollar, which is much less than you'd pay for an equivalent amount of meat....In addition to protein, beans are also high in folate, iron, fiber, and other nutrients."

Other real savings can be made by choosing where to shop. We were given the tip to buy our almonds in bulk at Costco or Trader Joe. They are so much cheaper there.

In the same way buying your wine at Costco means you can normally get three bottles for the price of two elsewhere. On the subject of saving money on wine, you will want to avoid the *very cheap stuff*. It may be bad for your health if loaded with sugar to make it palatable.

When purchasing eggs at the grocery store, select those that state the omega-3 content is high. Normally, they are only marginally more costly than the cheaper brands. Cheaper eggs may be from suppliers who have cut cost by feeding the hens animal fats, etc. Sally Fallon (ref.11 p.11) has a reliable comment:

"Organic eggs from hens allowed to feed on insects and green plants can contain omega-6 and omega-3 fatty acids in the ratio of one-to-one – but commercial supermarket eggs from hens fed mostly grain can contain as much as 19 times more omega-6 than omega-3."

Overcoming Stress
—Chapter 25

Our first teacher is our own heart.
Cheyenne Proverb

Without doubt stress can make arthritis worse. It also affects things like blood pressure.

As a recap, there are two types of stress—that brought about by one's reaction to external stimuli: and that self-induced by the way you eat. In this regard it is not only what you eat—but when you eat.

One can learn so much by *observing the evidence that is all around*. You too must know people with high blood pressure? In today's environment it is a common malady; and hence an opportunity to learn something new. Here are a few case studies to illustrate the point.

L.E. had given up his job to work fulltime in the retail business his wife had established. On one occasion he arrived at a factory, accompanied by his wife, to collect an order they had placed. He was not feeling particularly well that morning and needed to sit down while factory personnel loaded the product into their truck.

When the owner of the business asked if there was anything he could do to help, L.E. replied that his blood pressure was abnormally high and this was the cause of his being out of sorts. Then in the ensuing discussion between the couple and the owner, the latter was able to ask at an opportune time if L.E. had missed breakfast (they had arrived pretty early that morning), and if so could he get him anything in the hope it would make him feel better.

The owner was greatly surprised when L.E. replied that he never ate breakfast as that was one meal he could not handle early in the morning.

We move on to another person with high blood pressure, G.R. a college lecturer. Hers was so high; she had to take her medication with her wherever she went. She also had a weight problem, and desperately wanted to regain her slim figure. She had earlier discovered that skipping breakfast was easy to do. Therefore, she routinely skipped this meal each morning; only having a cup of coffee.

With regards her other meals they were not always as nourishing as could be because of the sugar and other stuff in the diet.

On to E.H. a grandmother who also missed out on breakfast: for the same reason as G.R. —she wanted to lose *a few pounds*. She too had excessively high blood pressure. In addition she ate the foods that have been identified as not being healthy. Salt was a favorite and it was used liberally on her food; way above the recommended daily allowance.

All in all there is a common denominator in the three cases above—that of missing breakfast. It is a bit of a mystery somehow that one can skip breakfast so easily. One can have a coffee and biscuit and feel as if you have had a meal.

However, the word 'breakfast' arises from *break the fast.* When you arise in the morning it can be anything between 12 and 14 hours since your evening meal—so the blood sugars are at fasting levels. Not to eat creates enormous internal stress within the body, as glycogen must be converted into glucose and as the body attempts to break down fat reserves. IMO, and based on an assessment of what we have seen around us, missing out on breakfast regularly eventually assists in causing high blood pressure.

Then too, later the overeating occurs, because of the famished feeling by lunchtime. This in turn creates more internal stress as adjustments are hastily and rapidly made from extremely low sugar levels to ingesting too much sugar.

As regards stress caused by external stimuli, Dr. Mercola (ref.17) warns that emotional stress causes chronic inflammation and increases bad cholesterol levels. It interferes with the body's natural cholesterol and cortisone producing ability. Stress creates enormous tension within the body: like being kept in a state of readiness to respond should something unexpected and terrible be about to happen.

What can aggravate stress is getting insufficient exercise. Physical exercise is good both for the body and the mind. Also, taking a vitamin supplement can help with stress. Dr. van der Merwe (ref.5 p.145) cautions that even *a marginal deficiency of folic acid can add to stress, and cause depression.*

It just keeps on cropping up that one should not eat those substances that can reduce the ability of the digestive system to absorb essential vitamins and nutrients.

Liberation From Depression
—Chapter 26

**Better fifty enemies outside
the house than one within.**
Irish Proverb

One of the penalties one *may have to pay,* as a consequence of having indulged in the sweet stuff, is depression. Think about it like this—that if by taking vitamins and supplements, one can obtain relief from depression, is it not logical to ask, "Whatever caused the absence of those vitamins in the first place—surely that is the source of the problem?"

On a visit to the Google website we found this helpful quote from the late endocrinologist John W. Tintera; given in the 1950's. He was quite emphatic regards the cause as you see:

"It is quite possible to improve your disposition, increase your efficiency, and change your personality for the better. The way to do it is to avoid cane and beet sugar in all forms and guises."

That is good news, really, for it supports the principle that by avoiding HFCS (not in mass-supply in Dr. Tintera's time), refined sugars and cereals, *one's health will improve.*

Although, as a consequence of previously eating sugar; your body may be so badly rundown that a *kick start* is necessary to restore it. Dr. Abrahamson (ref.3 p.63) has stated that Vitamins C and B12 and Niacin can help with depression. Adelle Davis (ref.4 p.7) has also stressed the importance of niacin in obtaining relief from depression, and we quote:

"Depression can be eliminated in a few hours by giving niacinamide."

Then too depression can be the result of a deficiency in certain minerals—as in this story:

R.T. shared how he had suffered from depression. He said he would be fine for long periods—then it would descend on him like a dark grey cloud. And suddenly too; as if he had been given an injection! He also told how he was addicted to candy and sweet stuff at that time.

Then rather unexpectedly his wife was contacted by a relative who had been on a visit to her doctor. This doctor had suggested that she should take magnesium as it was such an essential mineral supplement. When he heard the story from his wife he wondered if perhaps it might help him, and decided to give it a try.

To his surprise and immense relief his depression disappeared!

If you in turn decide to take magnesium oxide, remember it should be balanced with calcium in the ratio of one to two.

R.T.'s story was confirmed in Dr. van der Merwe's book (ref.5 p.133) where she states that calcium and magnesium are essential in the treatment of hypertension; leg cramps; tinnitus and vertigo—*including depression and anxiety conditions.* She goes on to say it is also used in the treatment of diabetes and hyperinsulinism.

Dr. van der Merwe (ref.5 p.146) has another indicator regarding the probable cause of depression when she says that too much omega-6 in relation to omega-3 can lead to depression.

(We have already mentioned that one of the methods to balance these fatty acids is by taking cod liver oil, along with the other oils and foods.)

Further supporting evidence to this fact was discovered on the website ZeroHedge.com (ref.36) in an article written by a contributing author; who writes under the pseudonym *George Washington* and posted on 1/21/13. In his excellent write-up he refers to the work of several doctors who are leading researchers on omega-3 fats. Here are a few brief and pertinent references:

To begin with, he quotes Olivier Manzoni and Sophie Layé as saying, "Our results can now corroborate clinical and epidemiological studies which have revealed associations between an omega-3 and an omega-6 imbalance, and mood disorders." They qualify their statement by adding that, "Additional studies are, of course, required."

The researchers go on to say that their results provide the first biological components of an explanation for the observed correlation between omega-3 poor diets, which are very widespread in the industrialized world, and mood disorders such as depression.

Next he quotes Dr. Northrup who writes, "One of the best ways to support brain health chemistry is by taking fish oil. Fish oil has been shown time and again to relieve mild to moderate depression."

According to Capt. Joe Hibbeln, M.D., Chief of Outpatient Services for the National Institute on Alcohol Abuse and Alcoholism (NIAAA), who is one of the world's leading researchers on omega-3 fats says, "These important fats *support the serotonin system;* may help reduce stress and lower your risk of all kinds of mental illness." He also says *the omega-3 fatty acids are essential to brain health.* Dr. Hibbeln's findings have been both compelling and encouraging.

The article ends by reporting that also heartening is the largest ever clinical trial, presented in 2009, which showed how fish oil may benefit half of all people with moderate to severe depression.

The author John Powell has written several books and in his most recent title *Happiness is an Inside Job* (ref.21 p.44) he stresses the importance of learning to relax, to exercise, *and to eat a properly balanced diet.* He confirms that a healthy body will "contribute greatly to a happy mind and a healthy spirit." He also stresses the importance of exercise, saying it is very difficult to feel depressed after a strenuous workout. Other authors have also written that a tired mind needs physical exercise.

Lastly, remember the importance of rest and sound sleep. The body heals itself when asleep. Lack of sleep can cause depression and the depression in turn will cause fatigue, exacerbating the problem, and so forth. And always live in the present moment—the past is gone: you cannot put toothpaste back in the tube! Then too, the future has not been yet given us. So learn to enjoy each moment and each day: following the guidelines for eating healthily.

Eliminating Constipation
—Chapter 27

One learns from one's mistakes.
German Proverb

Constipation is an embarrassing and personal subject. And because people do not speak about it: one is not aware of the extent of the problem. The large intestine or colon extracts water from the fine liquids passing through the small intestine. Constipation results when it absorbs too much. This can be brought about by drinking too little water, or through the system being adversely affected by sugar and refined and processed foods. Consider this case study:

C.C. had been a passionate lover of sweets and chocolates all his life. He was afflicted with constipation, and had suffered so intensely with the malady that he would be awakened in the middle of the night by pain in his colon. The way he handled the discomfort, whenever it occurred, was to go and sit in the kitchen and slowly drink water. Sometimes it could take as many as eight glasses before the pain subsided, or there was a bowel movement. On another occasion he told how he had to undergo a hernia operation as a consequence of constipation: the hernia being the result of the pushing.

When he luckily discovered the cause of the problem he said he changed to a healthier diet; excluding all sugars, and refined and processed foods. Fortunately, he persevered because although there was improvement along the way; it took 18 months for his system to become completely regular.

In his book, Dale Alexander (ref.2) states it takes from 12 to 18 months for the intestines to return to normal—once you cease eating the sugar, begin eating healthy foods, and improve your gut bacteria. He goes on to refer to the work of Dr. A. A. Fletcher (ref.2 p.198-199) who wrote a paper on constipation that was published in the *Journal of Laboratory and Clinical Medicine*. In it Dr. Fletcher mentions the work of Dr. R. McCarrison who put monkeys on a bacteria free diet, and one which was also high in starches.

According to Dr. McCarrison *their colon lost muscle tone and the membrane degenerated as a result.* He said the bowel changes in his experimental animals were structurally of the same nature as chronically constipated arthritics.

In his paper Dr. Fletcher also refers to Dr. R. Pemberton's research. What he did was to improve his patients' diets by restricting *inferior-type starches* like cake and candy. He then noted that their bowel actions improved for the better.

Finally, Dr. Fletcher makes it clear that more than one vitamin is deficient in the constipated person. But overall it is predominantly a deficiency of the B vitamins, which causes the bowel to break down and to lose its digestive action.

Adelle Davis in her book (ref.4 p.82) confirms the overall *sugar and starches theory* when she says that:

"Poor (waste) elimination can be corrected by a diet adequate in the B vitamins."

This all supports the fact that the sugar is the culprit; along with refined foods. It causes a deficiency in these vitamins (remember the body uses them up in metabolizing all the excess unadulterated or pure refined sugar—it has no option) and so the ability of the intestines to absorb the nutrients is impaired—and constipation results. Constipation is your body signaling you it is in trouble.

Referring to Dr. W. Davis in his book *Wheat Belly* (ref.9 p.66) we find similar sentiments when he confirms that when the intestinal lining heals and improves then better absorption of vitamins, minerals and calories once again become possible.

IMO a person suffering from constipation should abstain from, or seriously reduce dependence on laxatives as soon as possible. The system will heal and revert to normal once it is *treated correctly.* Do not be discouraged by the anticipated time it will take to become fully healthy—12 to 18 months may seem a long time; but from the moment you begin improvement starts happening! Consider this quote:

Wisely and slow;
they stumble that run fast.
Shakespeare

Becoming Slimmerer
—Chapter 28

In everyone's life, at sometime,
our inner fire goes out.
It is then burst into flame by an
encounter with another human being.
We should all be thankful for those
people who rekindle the inner spirit.
Albert Schweitzer

It has got to be the most discouraging thing when a person who is overweight: and who embarks on a program, in an effort to lose weight, through reduced eating combined with exercise— and instead of losing weight finds it being added on! Because they eat the wrong foods, they suffer intense gnawing hunger pains soon after a meal. And this continual suffering eventually makes it seem so in vain. No wonder so many people *throw in the towel* and then eat with abandon: and stop trying.

A good place to start if one has a real weight problem is by reading Dr. William Davis' book *Wheat Belly* and Dr. R. J.

Johnson's book *The Sugar Fix.* They explain the reason why the weight keeps being added on. It is as if the wheat has been developed to do this; and fructose has a similar bad effect. Armed with this knowledge one's confidence and purpose will be restored.

Also be very aware that *the low fat diet*—which has been given so much publicity in recent years—probably causes an increase in weight rather than the hoped for loss! Review this wise counsel from Adelle Davis (ref.4 p.31):

"Eating too little fat is probably a major cause of overweight…. Dr. Bloor points out that it would seem as if the body was speedily trying to produce the missing nutrients. This quick change makes the blood sugar plunge downward, causing you to be as starved as a wolf—the chances are you [then] overeat and gain weight… Fats are more satisfying [help you feel full] than any other foods. If you forego eating 100 calories of fat per meal, you usually become so hungry that you eat 500 calories of starch and sugars simply because you cannot resist them—unwanted pounds creep on."

If you are arthritic you do not want to be overweight; especially if it is in your spine or knees. An enlarged stomach places an excessive load on the spine and knees.

If you are overweight, say by five or 10 pounds—the next time you go to your grocery store pick up a bag of potatoes weighing the five or 10 pounds—and imagine it as that excess weight your spine and knees must support as you walk around. Conversely, losing that excess will help the knees.

But the situation is exacerbated if the sufferer does something stupid—even if from a lack of knowledge; and with the best of intentions. And about the *dumbest thing* anyone can do is to routinely skip breakfast.

If you skip breakfast then by lunch time your blood sugars are so low that you will *guzzle or wolf down* the food. Consequently, instead of losing weight—you add on the pounds. Adelle Davis (ref.4 p.102) has a scientific reason regarding cholesterol levels for why one should not miss meals: Note in particular her comments on the increase in weight when meals are missed:

"People frequently try to control weight by missing meals; the body uses a little food continuously and is overwhelmed by a day's supply coming at one time. In both animals and humans, *the blood cholesterol soars when only one or two meals are eaten daily*: it decreases when small frequent meals are obtained."

Here is an encouraging case study: B.P. was a chef at the Satara Camp in the Kruger national Park in South Africa. One morning, while doing the rounds at breakfast asking folk if they were enjoying their meal, he stopped at our table and engaged in conversation. Soon he sat down, and began telling stories of the various animals that groups of tourists had seen.

We were rather surprised when suddenly he asked if he could show us a photo of his former self. We were even more amazed when we viewed the obese fellow in the photo and compared it with the elegant fine looking specimen of a man sitting opposite us. In reply to being asked how he achieved the transformation he had this to say, "I had reached the point where I decided to do something about my grossly overweight situation. However, I very soon realized I needed a breakfast to get me through to lunchtime. But wanted to eat in such a way I could lose weight. Eventually what seemed to work well was having two scrambled eggs—nothing else! This got me through the morning and the weight literally fell away. Of course I *cut out the junk* at the other meals."

In support of what B.P. had discovered and put into effect; we came across an interesting article in the health section of the Daily Mail (ref.44). In it the reporter recounts the latest research at the University of Missouri. These researchers reported that a high protein breakfast of eggs is the best way to control appetite.

Another inspiring case study is from Adelle Davis (ref.4 p.211):

"A 76 year old woman, who had been in a wheelchair for years with arthritis, weighed 186 pounds."

The suggested meal plan for this person was: "Large servings of fish, fowl, or meat, with liver daily if she enjoyed it. A quart of milk, yogurt, cottage cheese and an egg daily, and a green salad at lunch and dinner tossed with a teaspoon of cold-pressed oil.......Now she is 40 pounds lighter and walks with a cane."

It is important to note that eating healthy foods is what helped the 76 year old woman to lose weight—no starvation plan—just eating scientifically! Another plus factor was the improvement in her arthritis—*from wheelchair to walking with a cane.*

Humorously, it can be said that in order to defeat *the fat man inside of one,* and who wants to take over—*you have to "trick him!"* To do so one needs an elementary knowledge of the workings of the body in relation to food requirements and the storage and processing of glucose. Then you can anticipate when food will be required by the body—and preempt or avoid those low sugar phases that make one ravenously hungry. Planning when and what to eat makes perfect sense.

People who lack a working knowledge and understanding of what goes on in the inside are at a distinct disadvantage, as in these instances:

S.M. and L.R. were two young men we observed sitting down in the food court in a mall, to have their lunch. What caught our attention was the similarity in their lunches. The one young man had a cola drink in a can, a chocolate bar and a white bread roll—the other a can of cola, a chocolate bar and an apple. *And that was lunch!*

Because of their age their weight had not as yet become a problem. But the certainty of the ill effects on their health long-term caused one to feel sad they had not been informed or educated about healthy eating, while at school or at home.

M.R. was a senior executive in a large corporation. He was rather conscious of the fact he was so overweight, and had tried several diets. One day at lunch he shared with colleagues his frustration at trying so hard and remaining largely unsuccessful. Therefore, at that particular lunch all he had served up was a large helping of fruit salad. He said that because fruit was so healthy, and he was not eating *rubbish* he hoped his latest attempts would bear results.

Sadly, M.R. did not have the benefit of Dr. Richard J. Johnson's research. We now know his efforts at reducing weight were in fact resulting in more pounds being added on—not to say anything of the hunger pangs M.R. would have felt a short while after lunch.

Dr. Johnson in his book *The Sugar Fix* (ref.8 p.82) warns repeatedly of the harm that is done to the body by ingesting large amounts of fructose. Doing so causes one to gain weight and interferes with the ability to lose weight—even if one attempts to cut calories, as stated above. Most men, as they advance in years, can develop a paunch. Dr. Johnson (ref.8 p.8) points out that this is caused by the sugars and particularly the HFCS in the diet. He says that eating fructose causes far more accumulation of abdominal fat—the worst kind—than the other forms of sugar, even if the same number of calories is consumed.

Dr. Mercola (ref. 17) in a newsletter regarding fructose has quoted from Dr. Robert Lustig's research—the following is a short excerpt:

"Dr. Robert Lustig, Professor of Pediatrics in the Division of Endocrinology at the University of California, has been a pioneer in decoding sugar metabolism, and his work reveals there are major differences in how different sugars are broken down and used.

For example: After eating fructose, virtually the entire metabolic burden rests on your liver. With glucose or most other sugars, your liver has to break down only 20 percent. The metabolism of fructose by your liver creates a long list of waste products and toxins, including a large amount of *uric acid, which drives up blood pressure and causes gout.*

Every cell in your body, including your brain, utilizes glucose. Therefore, much of it is "burned up" immediately after you consume it. By contrast, fructose is turned into free fatty acids (FFAs), VLDL (the damaging form of cholesterol), and triglycerides, which get stored as fat.

The fatty acids created during fructose metabolism accumulate as fat droplets in your liver and skeletal muscle tissues, causing insulin resistance and non-alcoholic fatty liver disease (NAFLD)[3] Insulin resistance progresses to metabolic syndrome and type II diabetes.

Fructose is the most lipophilic carbohydrate. In other words, fructose converts to glycerol-3-phosphate (g-3-p), which is directly used to turn FFAs into triglycerides. The more [fructose] you consume, the more fat you store!"

E.M. was a man who had formed the habit of using his bathroom scale each morning along with being conscious of noting what he ate. He noticed on several occasions that if he ate two or more pieces of bread during the day, it could mean an increase in weight the following morning of a full pound. By trial and error he came to understand the maximum he could eat was one slice of toast at breakfast—eat more than that and the weight would pack on.

The answer, as already mentioned, is to be found in Dr. William Davis' book *Wheat Belly* (ref.9 p.xi). He states that wheat today has been genetically modified to such an extent that it now *works against* a person; and makes them fat! He states that from his experience as a cardiologist, who sees and treats thousands of patients at risk for heart disease: he has personally witnessed *"flop-over-the-belt belly fat vanish"* when they have eliminated wheat from their diets. He says those overweight could lose as much as 20 to 50 pounds within the first few months.

To regain your ideal weight, and your health, means you must alter your diet to *exclude wheat;* and include those non-GMO foods that you know are healthy.

One final tip: to help with maintaining those blood sugar levels is that it makes good sense to have a snack—say, some almonds or occasionally a boiled egg—between meals. This keeps the sugar levels up and prevents that hungry feeling from developing, and gets you from meal to meal with ease.

Exercise And Rest
—Chapter 29

To know the road ahead
ask those coming back.
English Proverb

Just as in understanding how and what not to eat, applies equally to exercising.

Professor Possel, in a talk on heart attacks, spoke about the necessity of daily exercise. In it he suggested approaching the task in an intelligent manner. Meaning one should not do the body harm while attempting to firm up on muscle tone.

The example he gave was if you want to knock a nail into a piece of wood. You would not, for example, hold the nail in one hand and then with the other place the hammer on the nail. No! To get the nail to enter the wood one needs to raise the hammer and bring it down with "a blow" onto the nail.

In similar vein he suggested that when one goes jogging one places *hammer blows* on the knees, which can harm them in the longer term and as one ages. His suggestion, therefore, if one wanted to strengthen the heart (or other) muscles was to use an exercise bicycle. He saw this as the most efficient way to get fit.

In most research papers the necessity for exercise is paramount. For general health one needs to exercise—and the arthritic needs exercise for those joints. Our preferred method of exercising is walking; and it produces excellent results.

John Powell, in his book *Happiness is an Inside Job* (ref.21 p.49) states that what exercise does for us is to clear out from the brain and bloodstream the chemicals of tension. In effect exercise also promotes the production of chemicals that make us feel relaxed and peaceful, like the endorphins. And as mentioned in Chapter 26 above; it is very difficult to be depressed after a bout of vigorous exercise.

On the subject of protecting the knees, when selecting footwear ensure you purchase comfortable shoes. Those with a *shock absorber* positioned at the heal area are best—make sure they are comfortable to walk in.

As regards walking, learn to walk in such a way as to take the load off the knees. One person might walk in such a manner as to dig one's heels into the ground—in extreme cases the shock can reverberate up the legs and into the spine. Another will walk in such a way as to place one's foot almost horizontal on the ground; resulting in virtually no shock to the knees. If you do happen to be walking poorly, it will take no more than a month or so of practice to unlearn a bad habit.

On the topic of rest, the following are a few tidbits found along the way:

Switch off your TV at least 30 minutes before going to bed; and earlier for your laptop. You need a transition period where your mind can move from being highly active into a sleep mode. Read a little—and slowly—before putting out the light: something relaxing or contemplative; and not related to work or investments that will make the mind active during the night.

Then too do not shower or bath just before going to bed as it will make you fully awake. If you can, dim the lights so the body will begin secreting melatonin. And for those night time visits to the bathroom use nightlights, or a small flashlight, because putting on the main light will awaken you fully. This will make it difficult to fall asleep on returning to bed.

As well try not to have late nights. This old adage says it all:

Early to bed and early to rise;
makes a man healthy, wealthy and wise!

The advantages of a midday sleep or rest are incalculable. If you can manage a nap during your lunch hour then do so. If at home; then especially plan for a short sleep. In his book *The Blue Zones* (ref.26) Dan Buettner reports that it was found occasional napping was associated with a 12 percent reduction in the risk of coronary heart disease—but that regular napping, at least three days weekly—was associated with a 37 percent reduction.

Concerning insomnia, the worst thing one can do is to become anxious you are not sleeping and that you will be tired next day. Such anxiety will make you wide awake. Console yourself with the fact that if the body is really tired you will fall asleep. One author, many years ago, gave the example of British soldiers, who were being forced marched to Dunkirk at the beginning of the Second World War. They became so tired they fell asleep while walking. So the body will sleep if it really needs rest.   His suggestion was that if sleep was really eluding you, then to get up and read until feeling sleepy; and not to lie there fretting about it. But this only if your efforts to *get into sleep mode* before going to bed fail to work.

If awaking during the night, push your problems out of your mind. No amount of worrying will solve them—and they will still be there in the morning. All you do is rob yourself of the energy you will need to overcome them. If you do want to empty the mind of such worries—then fill it instead with prayer. And live in the present: especially at night.

Finally, taking calcium and magnesium with the evening meal will help achieve a relaxing good night's sleep. Taking the B vitamins during the day will also help. Make sure your diet contains sufficient potassium to keep those leg cramps away.

Red Flags From The Bible
—Chapter 30

There is a past which is gone forever.
There is a future which is still our own.
F. W. Robertson

Something new always seems to *keep popping up* in the Bible—
the more you read the more you appreciate how much there is:
even for your health.

In this regard, and as a start, you have to wonder at the
astuteness of the writings in the third book of the Bible, on
the subject of food. It would seem the author, Moses, had been
instructed that to effectively heal *or prevent* the onset of an illness, one should eliminate the *cause,* rather than be treating the
symptom.

For example, in this particular book of the Bible, the
Israelites are clearly forbidden to eat pork: as in this verse from
Leviticus:

Do not eat pigs.
They must be considered unclean;
Leviticus 11:7

Now before we continue it must be said that, today in our time, and regarding what is to be discussed: it is especially safe and hygienic to eat pork. But this was clearly not the case during early Jewish history.

In those days it was normal to have pigs or swine, wander around under the control of a herdsman. In addition there were often inadequate latrine facilities, with human feces sometimes found out in the open on top of the ground: and pigs would eat these wastes.

So the cycle for the tapeworm was unmistakably established. The pigs would eat the feces and the tapeworm parasite would make its way from the digestive tract into the pigs flesh. Subsequently, the pork would then be eaten by a human; and the parasite would lodge itself by attaching to the intestine wall: where it would grow as a tapeworm—and have the first choice of the best nutrients passing along the intestine.

The cycle is continued with the tapeworm depositing its eggs in what become the feces or human waste. In the meantime the tapeworm inside the person grows, seriously affecting the host's wellbeing.

By instructing the Jews not to eat pork, Moses ensured their safety and health was maintained: and consequently they enjoyed a better longevity than people in the neighboring nations who ate pork.

One can surmise that had sugar and white refined flour been around in the time of the early Bible; they too would have been mentioned and forbidden? As previously noted sugar consumption has only grown exponentially in the last 100 years—maybe one could say in the last 200. But even then remember it was not eaten in such great quantities as in more recent times.

Fortunately, in this regard there is more sound relevant advice to be had: for us in our situation. The first piece penned below is to refrain from eating anything which you know is bad and harmful: and then not to overeat.

> My child as you go through life,
> keep your appetite under control,
> and don't eat anything that
> you know is bad for you.

Sirach 37:27

> If you eat too much, you'll get sick;
> if you do it all the time, you'll
> always have stomach trouble.
> Gluttony has been the death of many
> people. Avoid it and live longer.

Sirach 37:30-31

Essentially the Bible wants what is best for you in so many areas of your spiritual and physical life—it even highlights the fact that a sound, healthy body is a veritable treasure. As is evidenced in this verse:

A sound, healthy body and a cheerful attitude
are more valuable than gold and jewels.
Nothing can make you richer or give you
greater happiness than those two things.

Sirach 30:15-16

Then again it reiterates the idea that some foods are definitely much better than others, and the implication is they are to be the preferred choice:

Any kind of food can be eaten,
but some foods are better than others.

Sirach 36:18

There is also encouragement regarding one's mental outlook. It says happiness makes for a long life. In this instance suggesting that to worry all the time is not good for one:

Don't deliberately torture yourself by giving
into depression. Happiness makes for a long
life and makes it worth living. Enjoy yourself
and be happy; don't worry all the time.

Sirach 30:21-23

The mission of this book is to explain how to regain and maintain bodily health.

Accordingly the readings above were provided as a source of encouragement. To show that even in the Bible your good health is desired and wanted. If you read the Gospels you will become aware of the number of healings done by the Lord Jesus, and that He wanted—and wants—to make people well again.

So it is appropriate to end with this quote from Jeremiah:

> I will make you well again;
> I will heal your wounds,
> I, the LORD, have spoken.

Jeremiah 30:17

Worthwhile Research
—Chapter 31

The person who can read, but
does not, has no advantage over
the person who can't read.
                                    Mark Twain

Reading good stuff is akin to applying fertilizer to the field of your mind. And the beauty of reading is you can learn in three weeks what it took the author a lifetime to discover.

However, before buying books it can be rewarding to search the internet. There are excellent search engines such as Google.com, Yahoo.com and Bling.com; and others. Wikipedia.org (ref.10) is a free Encyclopedia that is constantly kept up to date. It is full of outstanding resourceful information. On TV news a short while ago was reported the event of a teenage girl who had correctly diagnosed her illness through using the internet. The results having being confirmed by her doctor.

Unfortunately, just as in Louis Pasteur's time there will be a few doctors and other people with advanced education telling you harmful substances are 'good' for you! All we can say is think back to the era of the thalidomide babies who were born without limbs after their pregnant mothers had taken medication to combat morning sickness: medication developed by scientists and well educated people. If one listens intently to the business news programs you will frequently hear warnings from the FDA of drugs which have afterward been classified as harmful—in some cases being responsible for deaths in patients.

Consequently it does no harm to use your laptop to investigate the side effects of any medication which is prescribed to you. And be wary of those folk who tell you harmful substances will do you no harm—always look at the evidence around you!

There is no one person who has all the complete answers—that is why several books have been presented—and remember how medical statistics can be erroneously presented. As you progress in your research you will know who is reliable and when to be cautious—and of course you do not have to try everything that is recommended.

Regarding books, we are fortunate to have Amazon.com. Normally, every title you search for is available and you can get to read 10 percent of a book without making a purchase. Alternatively if you open their website and simply type in arthritis it is amazing the number of books on the subject that will appear.

Finally, it will help with our own ongoing research to hear from you—news of how eliminating sugar has improved your health and that of family and friends. Our email address is posted on the website ArthritisWise.com.

Preferred Reading
—Chapter 32

**A room without books is
like a body without a soul.**
Marcus Tullius Cicero

The total outlay for the suggested books below is probably less than the cost of a doctor's visit. To have these books on hand, and to be able to read firsthand these brilliant doctors and authors who have pursued in such a dedicated way, their dream of helping mankind by establishing the *cause of the illnesses* under review; and especially arthritis—is really a once in a lifetime opportunity. The outlay is a pittance compared to the knowledge one can gain.

Then too we now have Amazon.com where used books are available in excellent condition. Not only saving you money but making available books that, in some cases, are by now out of print.

"Body Mind & Sugar" by E.M. Abrahamson, M.D and A.W. PEZET (Ref.3)

This book surely forms the cornerstone of any small library devoted to restoring perfect health. If you are diabetic or suffer from hyperinsulinism, or arthritic, you really should buy this book, and study it from a medical perspective.

Just one example! It will explain in really simple terms the necessity for a five or six hour glucose tolerance test. Stuff you need to know when visiting your medical doctor.

It is so to your advantage to study the effects of sugar and certain foods and beverages on your blood sugar levels. It is an excellent introduction—written in layman terms—of how the body works regarding sugar. As far as we can ascertain Pezet was a former patient who, upon being cured by Dr. Abrahamson, wanted to assist in *getting the message out* and so volunteered to be the writer of the book.

The good news is that because of the body's ability to self-heal you should begin to notice an improvement in your health and well being after a few months by following the diets recommended by Dr. Abrahamson.

"Arthritis and Common Sense" by Dale Alexander (Ref.2)

Over a million copies were sold from 1954 through the 1980s. Therefore you can easily obtain a good used copy at Amazon.com for pennies and only pay the shipping. It has many case studies regarding the effectiveness of changing to a healthy diet.

His help given to arthritics is praiseworthy. He mentions cases of arthritics that left wheel chairs behind to walk again. He too has listed various diets that will help restore health.

"The Sugar Fix" Authors: Dr. R. J. Johnson with Timothy Gower (Ref.8)

Dr. Johnson calls a spade a spade and says it as it is. Furthermore he is Professor, Department of Medicine, University of Colorado, Denver. He speaks from a position of authority having verified his findings from his ongoing research.

Dr. Johnson provides much scientific and medical evidence from his research and analysis to support his contention that HFCS is harmful to the human body. Many doctors who formerly have said that sugar is not harmful—or is good for one—would do well to refresh on this excellent research and read Dr. Johnson's splendid work.

"Wheat Belly" Author: Dr. William Davis (Ref.9)

You will be angry when you realize how much has been *hidden from you*—and what has been done to our food: especially to that, which throughout history, has been known as *the staff of life*.

It is an essential read if you are overweight and need to regain your goal weight as set by your medical provider: or simply want to stay good-looking.

"Health & Happiness" by Dr Arien van der Merwe (Ref.5)

Dr. van der Merwe gives a most useful lesson in that throughout her book she is someone who continually treats the cause rather than the symptom. It is only natural we recommend her book as it was through it I found relief for meniere's disease—as is recounted in Chapter22. To be free from such an ailment is indeed a blessing.

There is so much else of real value in her book—as she promotes health giving supplements as opposed to taking medications, which as we know can have such harmful side effects. This book is an excellent reference and starting point when things go wrong with one's health.

"Sugar Blues" Author: William Dufty (ref.20)

This book is packed full of research that would take one many, many months to uncover. It is worth the money just to save the time. What is more it is necessary knowledge.

His presentation is to the point and easy to read. He pulls no punches in putting forward his assessment of the hazards of sugar.

"Let's eat right to keep fit" by Adelle Davis (Ref.4)

This is another of those books where the author focuses on the cause rather than the symptom. And the beauty of it is we have tried many of her solutions to so many ills. Her research provides a wealth of knowledge—the book is highly recommended as a read.

When you feel ill and do not know what is causing it—the resultant confusion robs one of happiness. Once you discover the cause your life becomes filled with purpose—you know the road to follow and this gives feelings of relief. The beauty of the book is that it is packed full of actual case studies where Adelle Davis achieved spectacular success.

Sally Fallon with Mary Enig, PhD "Nourishing Nutrition" (ref.11)

This book is considered essential reading for the arthritic seeking a cure and who wishes to remain healthy. For anyone in fact! The book is up-to-date with the latest research and there is so much of value. Hence the quotes used in the previous chapters and throughout the book highlight the credibility we placed on it.

While it contains many recipes and thus the book is 'sizeable'—the important literature is contained very neatly in the first 63 pages. These are considered a *must read.*

If you value yours and your family's health you will want to obtain this book.

Mercola.com (ref.17)

If you do nothing else you need to do yourself a favor and access this site and read the paper *The Cholesterol Myth That Is*

Harming Your Health by Dr. Joseph Mercola. The article could save you or a loved one much heartache in the future.

It explains in layman terminology what cholesterol is and how essential it is to your body. It also warns of the errors of some doctors in the way they treat cholesterol. Certain drugs that are presently being prescribed are actually potentially harmful and Dr. Mercola is in a position to comment on them.

Another article, relevant to our research on sugar, one should read is *Counting The Many Ways Sugar Harms Your Health* which is contributed by Dr. Nancy Appleton in May 2005, on Dr. Mercola's site.

As already mentioned in the previous chapters he has, among the many useful papers on his website, one on how to obtain sufficient potassium in your diet to avoid leg cramps.

Finally, on his website you can enroll for a free daily email newsletter to receive his articles and information concerning health issues.

Moving Your Goalposts
—Chapter 33

When I was sixteen, I asked myself: what if I
woke up every single day and I did everything
I could to change my life for the better —and
what if I did that for a week —a month
—a year!
Homeless to Harvard – Liz Murray

The author, John Powell, once asked in a talk, "Who were you thinking of when you had a toothache?" And then continued, "That's right—yourself and a dentist!"

In the same vein how can you be of help and assistance to others if you yourself are continually ill; or bedridden; or in-and-out of hospitals? You need your health more than you do money to be of use to others. John Powell (ref.21) has said that, "A sound body leads to a joyful spirit and a healthy outlook on life."

Be assured then that you are not being selfish or self-centered by taking care of your health—for with it not only are you a support to others: but you yourself will never become a burden. And the money you save in medical bills will be retained for your loved ones.

A good place to start is by being honest and admitting just how much you will feel deprived if you give up the sweet stuff. To what extent do you *crave sugar*—have you become addicted? If it is purely for pleasure—a frank admission helps you get in touch with your emotions and reasoning and is the first prerequisite to breaking the habit. Once in touch with those feelings: next you can figure out how to *change* them.

Concerning the potential loss in eating pleasure, or of having fun in a group situation where everyone is indulging; it helps to reflect first on this quote from Shakespeare:

**Things are rarely good or bad,
but our thinking makes it so!**

Shakespeare

Therefore, instead of feeling sad that one has to forego pleasure; you form the mental attitude that the stuff you are looking at is harmful—and if you eat it your health *will be* affected. Albeit slowly, but the damage will nevertheless be done. If you can change your thinking from *eating this will give me pleasure* to, *this is actually poison and will do harm:* you will become more resolute in saying, "No!"

However, if you are sorely addicted it may be a shock and harmful to your body to give it all up instantly. In that case consider this quote from Shakespeare and the story that follows:

> Wisely and slow;
> they stumble that run fast.
>
> Shakespeare

N.D. shared that he was relatively young when he got married. And it happened that his wife did not put sugar in her tea or coffee. He said that at the time he placed two heaped spoons in a cup of tea, and wondered how she managed to drink her tea without the sugar.

When he commented on her ability to go without the sugar; she made a most useful suggestion. To go slowly and cut out half a spoon at a time, getting used to the taste, until finally he would be able to drink his tea with no sugar.

N.D. said her suggestion worked, and the amazing thing about it was the tea tasted so much better without the sugar as one got to enjoy the aromatic flavors of the tea or coffee.

Another suggestion is to find substitute eating pleasures, especially when in a group situation where the others are all eating dessert. Try ordering or making up some fruit with natural yogurt. If the fruit comes out of a can remember to drain off the juices and discard, as it will contain sugar.

The longer you are free from the sugar habit, the more your 'taste buds' get restored. You will be truly surprised to find how succulent and sweet a natural juicy pear can be: or how delicious is a ripe orange and a bunch of fresh grapes. We can guarantee: so much better than a slab of chocolate.

Just make sure—if you have an excessive *sweet tooth,* which we all can relate to—not to overeat on fruit because of the high fructose content.

Remember you are on a mission to recover and preserve health—and by now you know what you are attempting is correct. This proverb inspires one:

**The future is not set, there is no fate
but what we make for ourselves.**

Irish Proverb

The third step is to visualize and keep on remembering the health that is on its way to you —and the happiness it will bring. Just as *love is a decision* so too is enjoyment.

Then too no one is infallible!

There will be times when one gives into temptation, or you are in a situation where eating food containing sugar is unavoidable.

Do not be hard on yourself. Rather think about how well you have done thus far and be resolute about trying again. Failing must and does happen to everyone because the following was penned so long ago:

**Our greatest glory is not in never falling
but in rising every time we fall.**

Confucius

Something that might help you understand what true happiness is—is to know that the opposite is pain and suffering through self-inflicted ill health! Do not wait until you lose your most valuable treasure. Be like Liz Murray above and make the decision and—*move your goal posts.*

The Health Prescription
—Chapter 34

Let food be your medicine
Hippocrates

Key Objective

To restore—and then to maintain—near ideal health through *eating as naturally as possible* those wholesome foods: meat; fowl; fish; whole milk, eggs and butter; with *plenty of* vegetables, and smaller portions of fruits and nuts.

Main Objective

Specifically, to avoid high fructose corn syrup (HFCS) and all forms of sucrose: no matter what guise it comes under. Avoid all delicacies and foods containing these substances.

To avoid refined flour, including breads, macaroni, pasta, etc., in addition to white rice and foods from which the nutrients and vitamins have been removed.

Secondary Objectives

Plan and space your intake of fluids so you do not drink with your meals. The exception is whole milk: but drink this in moderation at meal times.

Drink your red wine before your meals if possible—limit the amount you drink at actual meal times.

As a breakfast cereal use oats: make sure it has not been genetically modified.

Get quality sleep and rest; and relax every so often.

Place emphasis on exercise. Set aside a minimum of 30 minutes each day—but aim for one hour or more. Pray or meditate during this time. Alternatively, if needing to memorize something prerecord it and play it through earphones as you walk.

Plan your day to get a minimum of 10 minutes of sunshine; but preferably longer. Do some of your walking during the day time.

Monitor your intake of omega-6 type foods in relation to omega-3 type foods. Make baby lima beans; pinto beans; potatoes and broccoli (and the other nutritious vegetables) a frequent part of your diet.

Eat salads at mealtimes and / or some raw vegetables.

Take cod liver oil along with some of the essential oils such as flax and extra virgin olive oil. Include a vitamin E supplement.

Depending on your condition and needs, research what vitamins and supplements to take.

What to avoid

Avoid foods containing preservatives.

Avoid foods containing hydrogenated oils. It is in some peanut butters and potato chips.

Avoid—like the plague—all sodas and carbonated drinks—and especially all candy, sweets and chocolate.

Avoid fruit juices—these contain high levels of HFCS or sucrose and preservatives.

Avoid highly acidic fruits like lemons and limes. Limit the number of oranges you eat per week—as alternatives consider apples and bananas.

Avoid vinegar because of its acidic nature.

Avoid processed meats that may contain hydrogenated fats and preservatives such as MSG and nitrates. This may apply to some canned meats and foods.

Avoid honey if you are arthritic or have a sugar problem—it is almost totally concentrated fructose.

Avoid 'convenience' dinners that may contain HFCS, sucrose and hydrogenated oils. Remember *convenient* is not always best for health.

Avoid highly refined and processed breakfast cereals: especially those containing preservatives.

Avoid an excess of animal fats. While some animal fat is necessary in the diet, it should be eaten in moderation. Grass fed beef is best and generally costs much less at your farmers' market.

Avoid water containing fluoride. If purchasing bottled water be careful to establish what the supplier has added by contacting their customer service. Some suppliers add bicarbonate of soda, or sodium bicarbonate, to give the water a shelf-life. This will act as an antacid.

Warily assess those foods said to be 'all natural' or 'preservative free,' such as potato chips. Check to see whether hydrogenated oils or fats have been used in the preparation process.

EPILOGUE

A bit of fragrance always clings
to the hand that gives roses.
Chinese Proverb

Consider giving a copy of this book to someone who may benefit from it. The happiness and hope you can give to others by introducing them to the authors and researchers featured in this book are surely immeasurable? Especially today, when it is estimated there are over 50,000 books coming onto the market each month? No wonder these brilliant people have been buried in an avalanche of reading material.

You will have heard the expression—*What goes around, comes around.* And so it does. Therefore, by introducing others to the feasibility of a healthy lifestyle, and its benefits, you will eventually score directly. The more people who come to realize the folly of some of the stuff presented *as food,* the greater the chance of a public voice being raised in unison to bring about meaningful changes.

As a parting gesture; Dr. Ben Carson has said—*Knowledge can set you free.* So it is our sincere hope your newfound knowledge will set you free from the shackles of *deprived* health and *unwarranted* suffering.

In conclusion, as we anticipate you being happier—*and feeling that much better*—it is appropriate to end with the fuller version of the proverb given in the Foreword, viz.:

**Seeing is believing, but
feeling is the God's own truth.**
Irish Proverb

REFERENCES AND BIBLIOGRAPHY

1. Daisy Luther is a freelance writer and editor. Daisy writes about healthy prepping, homesteading adventures, and the pursuit of liberty and food freedom. Website: TheOrganicPrepper.ca Email: daisy@theorganicprepper.ca

2. "Arthritis and Common Sense" by Dale Alexander. Publisher: Simon & Schuster, as a Fireside Edition in 1981, Rockefeller Center, 1230 Avenue of the Americas, New York, New York 10020

3. "Body Mind & Sugar" by E.M. Abrahamson, M.D and A.W. Pezet. Publisher: Avon Books, a Division of The Hearst Corporation, 959 Eight Avenue, New York, New York 10017

4. "Let's eat right to keep fit" by Adelle Davis. Publisher: Unwin Paperbacks, Park Lane, Hemel Hempstead, Herts HP2 4TE, UK. © Harcourt Brace Jovanovich, Inc.,

5. "Health & Happiness" by Dr Arien van der Merwe. Publisher: Tafelberg Publishers, 28 Wale Street, Cape Town, South Africa, 8001

6. "The Primal Blueprint" by Mark Sisson. Publisher: Primal Nutrition, Inc, 23805 Stuart Ranch, Road, Malibu, CA 90265. MarksDailyApple.com

7. "The Blue Zones" by Dan Buettner. Publisher: National Geographic Society, 1145 17th Street N.W., Washington, D.C. 20036, U.S.A.

8. "The Sugar Fix" Authors: Dr. R. J. Johnson with Timothy Gower. Publisher: Pocket Books, a Division of Simon & Schuster, Inc. 1230 Avenue of the Americas, New York, NY 10020

9. "Wheat Belly" Author: Dr. William Davis. Publisher: Rodale Inc., 733 Third Avenue, New York, NY 10017

10. Wikipedia.org is a free Encyclopedia that is constantly kept up to date.

11. "Nourishing Traditions" Authors: Sally Fallon with Mary G. Enig, PhD. Publisher: New Trends Publishing, Inc. Washington, DC 20007 Website: NewTrendsPublishing.com

12. Wikiquote.org is part of Wikipedia, and is a free site that is constantly kept up to date

13. The Greatest Miracle In The World. Author: Og Mandino. Publisher: Fredrick Fell Publishers, Inc., Compact Books Inc., 2500 Hollywood Boulevard, Suite 302, Hollywood, Fl 33020

14. "Hand Washing." Author: Christine L. Case, Ed.D., Microbiology Professor at Skyline College Website: AccessExcellence.org/AE/AEC/CC/hand_background.php

15. DailyMail.co.uk/health: *Sugar is most dangerous drug of our time and should come with health warnings, says Dutch Health Chief,* Paul van der Velpen: Also at DailyPaul.com; Telegraph.co.uk; HuffingtonPost.co.uk

16. "World of Technology" Website: MyTechnologyWorld9. Blogspot.in

17. Dr. Joseph Mercola. 3200 W. Higgins Road, Hoffman Estates, IL 60169: Mercola.com

18. Ms. Margaret Durst. Margaret's Natural Health Blog, NaturalCowGirl.Wordpress.com

19. GraceLinks.org

20. "Sugar Blues" Author: William Dufty. Publisher: Warner Books, Inc. 1271 Avenue of the Americas, New York, NY 10020

21. "Happiness is an Inside Job" Author: John Powell. Publisher: Thomas More, an RCL Company, 200 East Bethany Drive, Allen, Texas 75002

22. "Help, Thank You!" Author: Ivan Cocks. Publisher: Ivan Cocks. www.Amazon.com

23. "Louis Pasteur" starring Paul Muni: It is screened on Turner Classic Movies (TCM), or you can purchase it direct from TCM.

24. "Mail on line – UK" Adapted from "Cooked" by Michael Pollan, Publisher: Allen Lane, UK

25. "The Irish Times", Thursday, April 25, 2013. www. IrishTimes.com

26. From NaturalSociety.com April 12th, 2013, Article by Anthony Gucciardi titled "Meet the Man Called 'Crazy' By Doctors Who Cured His Own Colon Cancer—story about Chris Wark."

27. Fox News – USA. http://www.foxnews.com/health/2013/07/09

28. Gerson Institute, 1572 Second Avenue, San Diego, CA 92101 Tel 619-685-5353 www.gerson.org

29. "Mediterranean diet is a combination deal say scientists," by reporter Genevra Pittman of Reuters. Website: Reuters.com

Source: the New England Journal of Medicine Website: nejm. org February 25, 2013

30. Chris Beat Cancer. A chemo-free survivor's health blog Website: ChrisBeatCancer.com

31. "Killing Cancer" by reporter Lori Johnson. CBN News Reporter, Friday June 21, 2013; Website: cbn.com

32. The Charlie Foundation; Website: CharlieFoundation. org

33. Author: Shari Rudavsky from The Indianapolis Star, owned by WBIR.com 1513 Bill Williams Ave., Knoxville, TN 37917. WBIR.com is owned by Gannett Co.

34. "Why butter is good for you" by Joanna Blythman and Rosie Sykes: The Guardian, Friday 12 July 2013: www.guardian.co.uk

34. EgglandsBest.com

35. RefreshingNews99.Blogspot.in

36. ZeroHedge.com

37. DrMirkin.com

38. Effect of cod liver oil on symptoms of rheumatoid arthritis. Advances in Therapy, 2002, Vol 19, Iss 2, pp 101-107. J Gruenwald, HJ Graubaum, A Harde. Gruenwald J, PhytoPharm Consulting, Inst Phytopharmceut, Waldseeweg 6, D-13967 Berlin, Germany

39. DrDavidBrownstein.Blogspot.com/2012/09/avoid-artificial-sweeteners.html

40. Chiropractic-help.com

41. QuackWatch.org

42. DrBass.com

43. The Gout and Uric Acid Education Society; Website: GoutEducation.org

44. DailyMail.co.uk/health/article-2306414/Another-reason-to-work-egg–lower-blood-pressure.html#ixzz2QBSK6sOz

45. The Holy Bible – Good News Translation

ALSO AVAILABLE
BY THE AUTHOR

Help, Thank You!
Amazing responses from
God to pleas for help

There are 42 stories in this book, from people who tell how the Lord God *'found them'* in their hour of need—and then helped them in a most profound way.